To Beth

With warm regards
+ appreciation —
Your Colleague,
Evelyn Nakano Glenn

Forced to Care

*Coercion and Caregiving
in America*

Evelyn Nakano Glenn

HARVARD UNIVERSITY PRESS

Cambridge, Massachusetts
London, England
2010

Library of Congress Cataloging-in-Publication Data

Glenn, Evelyn Nakano.
    Forced to care : coercion and caregiving in America / Evelyn Nakano
Glenn.
        p. ; cm.
    Includes bibliographical references and index.
    ISBN 978-0-674-04879-9 (alk. paper)
    1. Caregivers—United States.   I. Title.
    [DNLM: 1. Caregivers—United States.   2. Home Nursing—trends—
United States.   3. Home Care Services—trends—United States.   4. Social
Change—United States.   5. Social Conditions—United States.
WY 200 F697 2010]
HV1451.G64   2010
362.1'04250973—dc22   2009050638

Contents

Forced to Care

1

Who Cares?

As we enter the second decade of the twenty-first century, the United States faces an acute "care crisis." A spate of recent news articles and studies has sounded alarms about the large and growing gap between demand and supply in caregiving. The number of people needing care has risen much more steeply than the number of those available to provide that care. Nutritional and medical advances have lengthened average life spans so that the fastest-growing segments of the population are the oldest age groups—those in their seventies, eighties, and nineties—while medical advances, including drugs, medical devices, and treatment regimens, have extended life for people with chronic health problems and serious disabilities who might not have survived in earlier times.[1] Simultaneously, trends such as smaller families, geographic mobility, and high rates of employment among women have contributed to shrinking the pool of those who have traditionally provided informal care—wives, mothers, and other female relatives. As Mona Harrington describes the situation in *Care and Equality,* "We have patchwork systems, but we have come nowhere near replacing the hours or quality of care that the at home women of previous generations provided for the country."[2]

This trend has been clear since the 1970s as increasing numbers of women, regardless of marital and parental status, have entered the labor market. By 2000, 73 percent of women with children under age 18 were employed, a percentage that has remained fairly steady in the subsequent decade.[3] And, like other American workers, employed women put in long hours; they are among the overworked Americans, who, on average, work more hours and enjoy fewer vacation days and less paid leave time than workers in any other industrialized nation.[4] Extended work hours are making it difficult for Americans to meet their obligations to provide both economic support and care for dependent family members.

One reason the crisis has garnered public attention is that caregiving is no longer limited to poor families in which mothers have long had to work to support their families. Today, even relatively affluent middle-class families are experiencing a "time bind" and "stretch out" in their efforts to meet competing demands for income and caring.[5] Although a great deal of the concern about "work–family conflict" has been centered on child care, the fastest-growing aspect of the conflict is engendered by elder care responsibilities. Consider the following facts:

The average American couple now has more parents living (more than two) than children (fewer than two).[6]

Women now spend more years providing care for elderly parents (18) than for dependent children (17).[7]

In 2009, an estimated 43.5 million Americans were involved in caring for an aging relative or friend; about three-quarters of these caregivers had worked outside the home at some point since assuming care.[8]

The burden of elder care, as in other types of caregiving, falls most heavily on women, who constitute around 70 percent of informal caregivers. Women are not only more likely to be primary family caregivers for elderly kin, but they are more likely to care for those with more severe disabilities and to put in more hours of caregiving.[9]

Employed women are only slightly less likely to be primary care-givers compared to their age peers who are not in the labor force. Overall, about half of all employed women also care for a relative.[10]

Family caregivers who were employed full-time outside the home put in an average of 16 hours of unpaid care work, and those employed part-time put in an average of 21 hours; a sizable fraction of employed caregivers, whose elders are more severely disabled, put in over 30 hours a week.[11]

Women of color, especially African American women, are more likely to have to combine elder and disabled care with employment outside the home.[12]

Thus, although balancing employment and parental responsibilities remains a critical issue, the "new frontier" of work–family conflict involves care for elderly and disabled kin. This type of care poses unique challenges. Women who provide elder care are on average older than those who care for children; depending on the study, typical primary caregivers range from their mid-forties to their mid-sixties.[13] Older caregivers are more likely to have their own health problems. Additionally, with the current trend toward later age of childbearing, an increasing number of women—the so-called sandwich generation—are caring for both children and parents at the same time.[14] And, unlike care for non-disabled children, the intensity of both disabled and elder cares increases over time, rather than decreasing. A common pattern is for an employed woman to start off by providing small amounts of care and assistance but then to take on more and more responsibility as her parent becomes more frail and more disabled. Over time, the caregiving demands can become overwhelming.[15]

Many studies have documented high stress levels among family members who provide intensive care or who combine work and care for parents and disabled spouses and children. The demands of intensive care leave caregivers with little time or energy to look after their own well-being, so that their own health suffers. Numerous studies have shown that caregivers experience higher rates of heart disease, high blood pressure, diabetes, and depression.[16] Other studies have documented the detrimental economic effects of caring for elderly or disabled family members. One survey found that more than 50 percent of employed female caregivers accommodated by going to work late or leaving early, working fewer hours, giving up opportunities for upgrading skills or taking on special projects, turning down promotions, taking leaves of absence, choosing early retirement, or giving up work entirely.[17] A MetLife study estimated that employed caregivers who had to make a work adjustment because of caregiving responsibilities suffered a mean loss of $566,443 in wages, $25,494 in Social Security benefits, and $67,202 in pension wealth, for a total loss of $659,139 over the lifetime.[18] Another study found that women who engaged in care early in life were 2.5 times more likely to wind up in poverty than those who did not.[19]

Relatives, friends, and volunteers provide the lion's share (80 percent) of all home care despite the rigors and sacrifice required.[20] Still, they cannot meet the full caring needs of dependents, so there has been increasing demand for paid caregivers to substitute for or supplement family care. Paid home care is also allocated to women, who make up 90 percent of the care workforce.[21] Here again we find a gap between demand and supply. The U.S. Department of Labor reports that in 2006, 889,000 persons were employed in home health or personal care (undoubtedly an underestimation because many work in the informal job market) and estimates that these numbers will increase by more than 50 percent by 2016.[22]

Despite the purported shortage of available workers, wages remain low, with $9.22 an hour as the median nationwide in 2008, a level that is below the federal poverty level for a two-person household.[23] Medicaid home care benefits and state home care programs mandate low wages, often minimum wage, and also limit the hours of care that recipients can receive. Home care workers have to piece together a living by visiting and caring for several clients a day, often spending a lot of time traveling.[24] Additionally, home care workers usually get no paid vacation or sick leave, and many have no health insurance despite the high rates of on-the-job injury.[25] They are also specifically excluded from coverage by protective labor legislation such as minimum wage, maximum hour, overtime pay, and occupational health and safety laws.[26]

To be sure, paid care work offers its providers some intrinsic rewards, including the gratification of feeling useful and needed by their clients. Indeed, dedication to clients induces many care workers to remain on the job despite the financial sacrifices they may incur. Care workers may even do extra tasks or errands for their clients on their own time.[27] Still, the disadvantages of the work mean that home care work is too often a job of last resort, one that women who lack good options enter as a stopgap. Thus the ranks of paid caregivers are disproportionately made up of women (9 out of 10), racial minority women, and immigrant women.[28] The disadvantages of care work also account for the high rates of turnover, estimated at between 30 percent and 70 percent annually depending on location.[29] Many caregivers report that they enjoy their work and are devoted to their clients but are forced to find other jobs that pay better and offer benefits.[30]

This book is about the ideological and material foundations of the care crisis. It is grounded in the premise that the often untenable strains to which family caregivers are subject and the parlous situation of paid caregivers are closely intertwined and need to be examined together. The main thesis of the book is that the social organization of care has been rooted in diverse forms of coercion that have induced women to assume responsibility for caring for family members and that have tracked poor, racial minority, and immigrant women into positions entailing caring for others. The forms of coercion have varied in degree, directness, and explicitness but nonetheless have served to constrain and direct women's choices; the net consequence of restricted choice has been to keep caring labor "cheap," that is, free (in the case of family care labor) or low waged (in the case of paid care labor).

I put the social organization of care at the center of a number of important ethical, political, and economic dilemmas in American society and argue that the social organization of care has become preeminently a public issue, one that is integral to questions of economic and social justice, gender inequality, race inequality, class inequality, and citizenship rights. Let us start with some working definitions.

Caring can be defined most simply as the relationships and activities involved in maintaining people on a daily basis and intergenerationally. Caring labor involves three types of intertwined activities. First, there is direct caring for the person, which includes physical care (e.g., feeding, bathing, grooming), emotional care (e.g., listening, talking, offering reassurance), and services to help people meet their physical and emotional needs (e.g., shopping for food, driving to appointments, going on outings). The second type of caring labor is that of maintaining the immediate physical surroundings/milieu in which people live (e.g., changing bed linen, washing clothing, and vacuuming floors). The third is the work of fostering people's relationships and social connections, a form of caring labor that has been referred to as "kin work" or as "community mothering."[31] An apt metaphor for this type of care labor is "weaving and reweaving the social fabric." All three types of caring labor are included to varying degrees in the job definitions of such occupations as nurses' aides, home care aides, and housekeepers or nannies. Each of these positions involves varying mixtures of the three elements of care, and, when done well, the work entails considerable (if unrecognized) physical, social, and emotional skills.

By "social organization of caring" I refer to the systematic ways in which care for those who need it is allocated and how the responsibility for caring labor is assigned. Caring can be organized in a myriad of ways—in or out of the household, as unpaid family labor or as paid labor in the market. For example, caring can be provided within the home by a family member, friend, or community volunteer without pay or by a servant or home care worker for pay. It can be done in more collective settings such as community day care centers by a combination of volunteers and paid staff or in an assisted-living facility or a nursing home by paid employees. Furthermore, the care may be arranged and overseen by the care receiver, the care receiver's family, a non-profit entity, a government agency, or a profit-making company. Caregivers can be remunerated by care receivers or their relatives, by private insurance, or by government agencies. These arrangements are not mutually exclusive. All these forms exist simultaneously in contemporary societies.

However, the particular mixture and balance of paid and unpaid, commodified and non-commodified, and private and public forms have varied across time and place, reflecting a society's economic structure, prevailing beliefs, political systems, and cultural practices. In the United States the social organization of care has been characterized by reliance on the private household, feminization and racialization of care, devaluation of care work and care workers, and abnegation of community and state responsibility for caring. The persistence of these characteristics, despite (or perhaps because of) the frequent lip service given to the spiritual and moral qualities of caregiving, is rooted in fundamental philosophical principles, social structures, and cultural practices that have survived (in somewhat altered forms) since the early republic. For this reason, an examination of historical continuity and change in these structures, beliefs, and practices is essential for understanding the material and ideological underpinnings of the contemporary social organization of care. Such an analysis is also crucial to identifying contradictions and fault lines that might be exploited to transform the way care is organized in our society.

The final concept is that of coercion, which I define as physical, economic, social, or moral pressure used to induce someone to do something. In the case of caring, two specific forms of coercion are particularly relevant. The first form is status obligation. As described by Alvin Gouldner, status obligations are duties assigned to all those in a given status, for example, wife, mother, daughter. Gouldner notes that status obligations "may require an almost unconditional compliance in the sense that they are incumbent on all those in a given status simply by virtue of its occupancy."[32] A status obligation can be contrasted with the norm of reciprocity, in which an obligation is incurred as a *debt* for gifts and services that one has received. Status obligation can also be contrasted with contractual obligations that are incurred as a result of voluntarily entering into an agreement to provide services in exchange for pay or other considerations. Scholars since the time of the nineteenth-century anthropologist Henry Maine have argued that as Western societies modernized, they shifted from reliance on status relations to contractual relations. In this view, market relations have been more or less completely contractualized, but family and kin relations have remained "premodern" in that status obligations remain in force.[33] I will argue that status categories such as race and gender continue to shape both market and kin relations. Consequently, women are charged with a triple status duty to care, on the basis of (1) kinship (wife, daughter, mother), (2) gender (as women), and (3) sometimes race/class (as members of a subordinate group).

The second form of coercion is racialized gendered servitude, by which I mean a labor system in which one party has the power to command the services of another. In some instances, the power is de jure, in that one party is recognized by law as having a property right in the person and/or labor of the other. Slavery, indentured labor, and debt bondage are prominent examples of racialized gendered servitude that have at one time or another been legally recognized in the United States. In other instances the power is de facto, in that it grows out of marked inequality between parties, whether economic, physical, or social. Contemporary examples of inequalities that have fostered servitude include undocumented immigrant workers in sweatshops in U.S. territories, impoverished child servants in many parts of the world, and women trafficked into sex work or domestic services. I use the qualifier "racialized gendered" because the lines that distinguish those who command services from those who provide them are often those of race and gender (e.g., white/black, male/female), and ideologies that support the rights of those who command others are framed in terms of natural differences between races and genders.

As we will see in Chapter 2, these two traditional forms of coercion were "modernized" and reestablished during the country's transition from a predominantly agricultural society to an industrial economy. This shift took place over the course of the nineteenth century and occurred unevenly across regions and sectors of the economy. In two distinct but intersecting threads in the history of caregiving, the first trajectory is that of a "free-labor" system that developed in the industrial and advanced sectors of the economy. The households of workers in free-labor sectors came to be characterized by a gender division of labor in which men were primarily responsible for breadwinning through outside employment in the labor market and women were made responsible for housework and caring in the "private sphere" of the family. The second trajectory is that of unfree-labor regimes that survived into the early twentieth century in peripheral regions of the country, especially in primary sectors of the economy such as agriculture and extractive industries. In these sectors, households relied on outside employment from both men and women. The labor markets in these sectors were structured so that men of color were tracked into and confined to low-wage, non-mechanized labor, and women of color were tracked into domestic service and caring labor for more privileged households. The imprint of these historical formations can still be seen in contemporary patterns and practices in both unpaid and paid caring labor.

In Chapter 3, we will examine how these trajectories intersected in class, race, and ethnic relations among women. During the late nineteenth and early twentieth centuries, as part of its nationalist aspirations, the United States sought to reform groups and individuals who were seen as deviating from "American ideals" and thereby as threatening national unity. These reform efforts opened up opportunities for elite and middle-class women to extend their caring activities into the public realm as agents of "female reform." Their role became that of educating subaltern women in the ideals and practices of female domesticity and caring. Three female domestication efforts will be examined: the training of Native American women in the Indian boarding school system, the rehabilitation of women inmates in female reformatories, and the "improvement" of non–Western European immigrant women through so-called Americanization programs. These efforts shored up prevailing ideological constructions of women as carers and moral touchstones of the family and ultimately of the nation. Importantly, these case studies demonstrate that reshaping subaltern women to fit middle-class norms of female caring was integral to efforts to control racial, ethnic, and lower-class "others."

Chapter 4 delves into the roots of the inequitable burden that women bear for unpaid care labor. We will develop the concept of caring as a status duty for women and examine the role of the state in defining and enforcing this obligation. I focus on two areas in which the state historically articulated and enforced women's obligation to care: marriage and family law, which codified wives' duty to provide domestic services, including nursing care, and social welfare provisions for dependent disabled individuals, which presumed that family members, particularly wives and mothers, had primary responsibility for providing unpaid care. Despite nineteenth- and twentieth-century modernizing reforms, law and social policy have continued to affirm the principle that the family, and not the community or the state, bears primary responsibility for meeting dependency needs, and that family members (parents, spouses) are obligated to provide care for other family members.

Paid care work has long been treated as though it was an extension of women's unpaid domestic labor rather than as a legitimate form of wage labor with its own standards, training requirements, and pay scales. In Chapter 5, we will focus on the exclusion of home care workers from legal protections provided by the federal Fair Labor Standards Act and the Occupational Safety and Health Act. Justifications for excluding home care workers from standard protections have historically been framed in two ways: first, the need to protect the privacy of the household so that it can function as a haven in an otherwise heartless world, and second, the household employer's entitlement to the services of domestics servants and caregivers so as to ensure that members enjoy the comforts that a home is intended to provide. In contrast to explanations for the exclusion of home-care workers that focus on the first set of justifications, namely the location of home-care work in the private household, I will argue for the equal significance of the second set of justifications, namely the quasi-property rights that employers enjoy with respect to servants. An examination of U.S. immigration laws that allow entrants holding certain kinds of visas to be accompanied by household servants further reinforces the conclusion that the exclusion of home-care workers from protections provided to other categories of workers has rested on its dual construction as an aspect of private household family relations (therefore governed by principles of altruism and status obligations) and as an extension of earlier relations of indenture and slavery (therefore governed by principles of property ownership).

Chapter 6 sheds light on how contemporary neoliberal economic and political trends have contributed to the caring crisis. We have witnessed the confluence of three trends that have intensified the demands and difficulties of caregiving and have exacerbated the coercive factors that impinge on both informal and low-paid care work: first, the devolution of care (especially acute health care and nursing) back into the private household; second, the dismantling of welfare programs for poor mothers so as to compel them to undertake low-wage jobs in the labor force; and third, the neoliberal economic restructuring that has displaced people from traditional means of livelihood in poorer countries that make up the global south, thus sharply accelerating female labor migration to the United States and other rich countries in the global north. We will examine the impact of these developments on the care labor of three groups most affected: white middle-class women, poor single mothers, and immigrant women from the global south.

Taken together, the historical accounts and contemporary developments demonstrate how caring labor has undergone continuous reorganization in concert with changes in political economy. Despite the shift of care from home to the market and back again and from unpaid to paid and back again, race, gender, and class have remained central organizing principles of care labor. As a result, care labor remains an arena where coercion holds sway and where full freedom and citizenship are denied.

Assuming that legal and economic coercion is not a good basis for quality care and that the true needs and interests of care receivers, family caregivers, and paid care workers must be addressed in order to create a caring society, in Chapter 7, we will look at the ways in which care work needs to be rethought and reorganized. Rethinking care involves dismantling the dichotomies that have delimited care: private versus public, love versus money, and altruism versus self-interest. Confining care to one side of these dichotomies (private, love, altruism) has obscured the public function that care labor serves and has masked its central place in the economy. Rethinking care also requires attention to the needs of care receivers and caregivers and a balancing of the right to receive needed care with the right to provide care without excessive economic penalties or sacrifice of well-being. We will also examine alternative goals and strategies for addressing the care crisis and the extent to which they mitigate the coercive structures that have disadvantaged care workers.

Together with other advanced industrial countries in the world, the United States faces an unprecedented challenge of ensuring that its growing numbers of elderly and disabled citizens receive the care they need and deserve. Addressing this issue demands a fundamental rethinking of care that will require us to uncover and analyze the material and ideological roots of the present care system and to understand how the system has come to rely on the exploitation of women's labor and the denial of equitable benefits and entitlements. Exploitation has been made possible by multifarious forms of coercion, ranging from personal moral persuasion to the force of impersonal legal doctrines, from internalized feelings of obligation to external constraints of the labor market. By tracing the multiple strands of coercion, I aim to expose the social inequality and denial of social citizenship that lie at the heart of our present system of caring.

2

Caring for One's Own and Caring for a Living

During colonial and early republican history, the United States was largely an agrarian society in which households constituted the basic economic units for both production and reproduction.[1] Most households grew and processed their own food and manufactured many of the goods consumed by family members. They were also responsible for social reproduction, that is, maintaining their members both on a daily basis and intergenerationally. Labor was divided along both gender and generational lines. However, the divisions were relatively fluid, and productive and reproductive labor were not sharply differentiated. Wives were responsible for cleaning, cooking, watching over children, and nursing members who were ill—but they were simultaneously engaged in processing and preserving food and making clothing, candles, soap, and other household items. Husbands were primarily responsible for outdoor work, such as plowing fields, planting, and harvesting, but helped with spinning and weaving and also were involved in supervising children and training sons in farm tasks. Children were also expected to contribute their labor, with sons assisting fathers and daughters assisting mothers.[2]

To be sure, women's economic independence was severely restricted by the common-law doctrine of coverture carried over from England. Upon marriage, a woman's legal identity was subsumed by that of her husband. Economically, this meant that a household's assets and labor were held in the husband's name. A wife's labor was owned by her husband, and any products or cash realized from the sale of her labor or its products belonged to him. At the same time, because wives were considered helpmates, they could act as deputies to their husbands, carrying out all manner of transactions, negotiating with merchants or sellers, and collecting and paying debts. As Laura Thatcher Ulrich has noted, no business activity was ruled out for wives as long as it was understood to be for the good of the family.[3]

Moreover, up until the 1790s, it was not uncommon for single women and widows, and even some married women, to run businesses on their own account. In port cities, such as Charleston, South Carolina, and Newport, Rhode Island, which had sizable transient populations, women were active in the service economy. They ran boarding houses, taverns, and shops and took in laundry and tailoring. In New York City, some women, married as well as widowed and single, engaged in complex trading activities, buying and selling commodities. In Philadelphia, female heads of middling households, mostly widowed and single, acted as proprietors running small businesses, while women from poor families made livings as hucksters, vendors, and washerwomen.[4]

The mid-eighteenth century marked a high point for independent female entrepreneurship. Toward the end of the eighteenth century and the early decades of the nineteenth, independent female entrepreneurship declined. Governments and courts made it more difficult for single and widowed women to make contracts and for married women to maintain separate estates by enforcing coverture principles.[5]

The hardening divide between men's and women's economic activity was mirrored in political rhetoric. Before the American Revolution, when subjectship rather than citizenship defined people's relationship to the state, dependence was a common condition, one shared by most men and women. In contrast, independence was an unusually privileged status, reserved for those who had sufficient property that they could live without laboring. Such persons were described as "being independently wealthy" or "having an independent means."[6] Economic independence was in turn thought to be a precondition of political independence. It was believed that only those who did not have to rely on another for a living could be free to act for the common good. Thus, when representative government was established in the United States, property ownership was made a prerequisite for suffrage, disqualifying not only married women, but also non-propertied men.[7]

Broadening the meaning of independence to include those who worked for a living was indeed a revolutionary concept. In making the case for breaking away from the British crown, supporters of revolution stressed the importance of independence, arguing that liberty required independence and that being made dependent was to be reduced to being a slave. The divide between independence and dependence was drawn along race and gender lines. White men, by virtue of their gender and race, were deemed to be categorically independent, whereas non-whites and all women were categorically dependent.[8]

Proponents of equality among white men drew on a Lockean theory of natural rights. According to Locke, men had been equal in a state of nature. They came together to form a social compact in which, in exchange for giving up some personal rights, they gained government protection to the rights to life, liberty, and property. Rosemarie Zagarri points out that although the notion of a compact implied corresponding duties that accompanied freedom, "when Americans translated Locke's theory into practice, they tended to minimize the importance of duties and enhance the importance of personal autonomy and individual choice."[9] What made (white) men free was ownership of their own labor, which they could voluntarily contract. This schema excluded not only white women but also African Americans and Indians, who were viewed as lacking the capacity to contract their own labor. It thereby ignored subgroups such as single women, free blacks, and "civilized" Indians who theoretically could contract their own labor. Instead of changing their conceptions to take into account these exceptions, political leaders helped to erect legal barriers to hobble the ability of women, free blacks, and Native Americans to earn and demonstrate independence.

Zagarri notes that some writers agreed that women also had rights, but asserted that their rights differed from those of men. In place of Lockean natural rights, these writers turned to philosophers of the Scottish Enlightenment who rejected social contract theory and assumed the necessity of social hierarchy to maintain social order. These thinkers drew on a Protestant natural law tradition that "emphasized duty over liberty and custom over contract" and equated rights with duties rather than with political liberty and personal autonomy. For example, a woman writer, Hannah Crocker, opined that a woman's rights consisted in nurturing her children and taking care of her husband: "It must be women's prerogative to shine in the domestic circle," she wrote, "and her appropriate duty to teach and regulate the opening mind of her little flock. . . . The surest foundation to secure the female's right, must be in family government."[10] Another writer, a Miss M. Warner, a self-proclaimed champion of the "Rights of Woman," related what she considered women's rights: "to cook delicious meals, to share in her husband's grief, to nurse him when he is sick."[11]

As these excerpts reveal, a critical aspect of late eighteenth-century ideological currents was the gendering of public and private spheres and the redefinition of the moral values associated with each. In classical Western political theory, the public realm was where men came together, suspending their selfish interests, in order to act for the greater good. The private realm, where women, children, and slaves were confined, was associated with dealing with mundane matters and the furthering of self-interest.[12] Revolutionary-era rhetoric reinforced the public–private divide but elevated the morality of the private realm above that of the public, depicting the home as the original seat of virtue.

This domestication of virtue provided openings for women to claim a special kind of gendered citizenship. Joan Gunderson identifies two related discourses that emerged in the late eighteenth century to claim a civic role for women as mothers. The first was the discourse of "Republican Motherhood," a name given by Linda Kerber to a strain of thought that linked women's private virtue to men's public virtue.[13] According to Gunderson, "Philosophers, novelists, and poets sentimentalized a mother's influence over a child and invested it with the power to shape morals and patriotism. Love of family was the model for loving one's country." As women took this message to heart, they embraced Republican Motherhood. Mothers would shape good citizens for a new republic."[14]

A second discourse was that of Evangelical Motherhood, "a less political, more private vision" than that of Republican Motherhood. In this discourse, "women would shape their families into committed Christians." In contrast to the ideology of Republican Motherhood that assumed that the home served a public function, Evangelical Motherhood "was premised on the ideal of the home as an 'island of purity' that needed to be kept separate from a corrupt world."[15]

Although Republican and Evangelical Motherhood held contrasting assumptions about the public sphere, this difference was overlooked by most American women, who focused on their common emphasis on domesticity and motherhood.[16] Gunderson avers: "By 1790 the two main elements of the new norm—women as dependent nurturer and moral guardian—were widely accepted. Ideas of female piety converged with an understanding of virtue as a moral (emotional) sense and the sentimentalization of domestic relations. . . . Over time, the new nation obliterated the traditional flexibility allowing women to assume a wide variety of roles by converting domesticity from a role into a biological trait."[17] Importantly, both Republican and Evangelical Motherhood were racialized concepts that left poor people, Native Americans, and African Americans outside the dominant standards of ideal family and gender relations.

Before industrialization, care labor was integrated into the domestic economy. Women were primarily responsible for caring, but they also contributed to the family's livelihood by producing goods for family consumption and for barter or cash. It was understood that both husbands' and wives' labor was essential to the household economy. Even in this period, however, men's and women's labor contributions were calculated differently in that under coverture, money or property acquired through a wife's labor belonged to and was controlled by her husband. Nonetheless, a wife's unpaid labor was commonly understood to have economic value. This basic understanding began to change with the development of republican ideals of separate male and female spheres and responsibilities.

The Market Revolution and Early Industrialization

The conception of wives' unpaid labor as categorically different from men's labor became more pronounced with the growth of the market economy and industrialization in the United States. Historians have referred to the economic changes that occurred in the late eighteenth and early nineteenth centuries as a "market revolution." By this they meant the transition from mainly local markets, operating according to traditional customs and status relationships, to a national market, governed by impersonal economic factors such as supply, demand, and price. As John Lauritz Larson describes the shift: "After the market revolution, money alone mobilized goods and people, no matter how grand or mean the owner of the purse."[18] Whereas before the market revolution goods were custom made, production in the nineteenth century increasingly focused on ready-made (and therefore standardized) goods. Master craftsmen who earlier had employed skilled journeymen turned to less skilled or cheaper labor (apprentices, women, blacks) to increase output.[19]

Journeymen responded to heightened competition for jobs and declining wage levels by forming workingmen's associations and unions. In addition to speaking out against predatory practices in banking and financial markets, workingmen's groups called for a "living wage," one sufficient to support a man, his wife, and his children.[20] Such a wage, they claimed, was necessary for working men to maintain their standing as heads of households and to fulfill their obligations as family breadwinners. In his study of New York City male workers involved in unions and worker associations in the period from 1800 to 1840, Joshua Greenberg argues that family and household relations and identities as husbands and fathers were as central to their activism as their workplace relations and identities as workers. In speeches and writings, organized workers frequently evoked home, wives, and children as the inspirations for their striving. Workingmen's newspapers featured stories not only about workplace issues but also about family and community concerns. They regularly reported on significant family events, announcing the birth of children, marriages, and bereavements.[21]

According to Jeanne Boydston, "In the context of a society in which men's ownership of the family labor time had already been transformed into a perception that men were the only laborers in the family economy, the 'family wage' ideal worked to reinforce the invisibility of the wife's contribution." The ideal also incorporated the ideal of female domesticity, contrasting women's unpaid household activities and men's wage labor:

> Workingmen's newspapers contrasted the "odious, cruel, unjust and tyrannical system" of the factory to the . . . "calm quiet retreat of domestic life." . . . Early trade unionist William Sylvis waxed sentimental about the charm of women's mission: "To guide the tottering footsteps of tender infancy in the paths of rectitude and virtue, to smooth down the wrinkles of our perverse nature, to weep over our shortcomings, and make us glad in the days of our adversity, to counsel, and console us in our declining years."[22]

Despite the rhetoric, married women's labor continued to be crucial for their families' living standards. Nancy Folbre notes: "The wives of farmers, merchants and craftsmen participated in family enterprises. Many women took in boarders and lodgers, exchanging household services such as cooking and cleaning for money. Housewives provided their own families with an even wider range of domestic services—meal preparation, laundry, child rearing, care of the sick and elderly, household management, and general nurturance."[23] Women and children in poorer families scavenged. In urban areas they foraged for fuel, food, and old clothing; in rural areas and the outskirts of cities, they gathered bullrushes used to cane chairs, cattails to stuff mattresses, and straw to make brooms.[24]

Simultaneously, the expansion of the market economy and accompanying political and social changes increased opportunities for single women to earn outside the home. The first factories and mills in early nineteenth-century New England recruited the most readily available labor force, young single women, primarily from farm families. This period also saw the spread of public schooling designed to ensure an educated citizenry.[25] There were regional variations in the gender composition of school teaching, but especially in the Northeast and many parts of the Midwest, elementary school teaching became increasingly feminized during the nineteenth century, at least in part because women could be hired for a third to half the salaries of male teachers.[26] Whether in factories or schoolhouses, single women's employment was considered short term, to be abandoned after a few years for marriage. Moreover, their outside employment was always contingent. If their services were needed at home, for example if a parent fell ill and needed care, they were expected to quit their jobs and return home to nurse that family member.[27]

Despite the critical contributions that wives' and daughters' labor made to the family economy, the concept of a family made up of a male earner employed outside the home and wife/mother engaged in unpaid reproductive labor at home became the dominant ideal. The public–private distinction and the notion of separate male and female spheres that emerged in the eighteenth century among elite households spread to middling families and skilled tradesmen and their families.

This conception reflected the growing spatial separation of work and family life, which increasingly took place in different locations. For example, according to Katherine Osburn, in 1790 almost all New York City artisans had workshops attached to their homes; by 1840 two-thirds of them lived and worked in separate places.[28] Relations between journeymen and masters/bosses became less familial because they no longer lived together.[29] Conversely, relations between husbands and wives came to be viewed less in terms of economic exchange (husbands' support for wives' services) and more in terms of mutual affection, companionship, and emotional support. The home and the market (private and public) came to be understood as distinct and bounded spheres that operated according to completely different principles. According to the emerging ideology, the market exalted impersonality, competition, independence, and self-interest, whereas the home/family valued personalism, harmony, dependence, and selflessness. The private household came to be viewed as a refuge from the public realm, a necessary sanctuary from the stresses and strain of the workplace.

Joan Gunderson argues that the actual content of women's work changed less than the ideological meaning of their activities: "Married women did not stop making clothes, candles, or butter, but the meaning of these tasks changed. They were now symbols of women's domesticity, nurturing, and virtue. Women's production was no longer defined as 'work.' Women were seen as dependent consumers in a market economy."[30] Jean Boydston emphasizes that the rise of the cash market reshaped both men's and women's perceptions of "women's work." She notes: "Women's private diaries and letters suggest that they also discounted their contribution to the economic needs of their families. During this period, for example, some wives began to draw a distinction between the labor of cooking, cleaning, and washing, and the other work they performed—particularly work that created goods associated with the market, whether the goods were actually sold or not." She cites an entry in the diary of Lydia Almy, the wife of a mariner in Salem, Massachusetts, "who wove, attended to livestock, made cider, carted wood, tanned skins, took in boarders, and sometimes worked in the fields, nevertheless recorded in her diary that she was 'in no way due any thing towards earning my living which seems rather to distress my mind knowing that my dear husband must be exposed to wind and weather and many hardships whilst I am provided for in the best manner.'"[31]

The Housewife and the Breadwinner

Industrialization was heavily implicated in the final shift of production away from households and into factories, shops, stores, and offices. The first phase of industrialization in the early nineteenth century had focused on centralized production of consumer goods, some of which had previously been made at home—cloth, clothing, shoes, soap, and candles—and others that had been fabricated in small workshops— paper, books, newspapers, furniture, clocks, bricks, guns, and ammunition. Toward the middle of the nineteenth century, mechanized farm equipment began to transform agriculture. Farmers could cultivate larger plots of land and increase their yield of market crops. The establishment of a new type of corporation, the private bank, which issued its own currency, provided capital for investment in large-scale enterprises, while the development of turnpikes, canals, and transportation systems made it possible for manufacturers and farmers or their agents to transport locally made goods and locally grown produce to towns and cities throughout a region.[32]

The Civil War ushered in a second phase of capitalist industrialization. Late nineteenth- and early twentieth-century industrialization was on a much larger scale and concentrated on capital goods, that is, goods that added to productive capacity, for example, railroad equipment, factory machinery, and construction equipment. During the 1860s and 1870s the completion of transcontinental railroad lines and telegraph networks linked local producers of raw materials, manufacturers, and growers to national markets. In this second phase of industrialization, individual proprietorship gave way to new forms of ownership, corporations, monopolies, trusts, pools, and holding companies. These organizational forms permitted vastly larger-scale production while limiting liability for owners and investors.[33]

Capitalist industrialization severely reduced opportunities for independent livelihood. By the 1860s, wage earners had come to outnumber those working on their own account, and the ratio of wageworkers to independent producers continued to grow over the following decades.[34] Moreover, it was becoming clear that wage earning was no longer a temporary way station on the path to independent entrepreneurship but rather a long-term "career." To be sure, many of the new waged positions offered substantial remuneration and opportunities for advancement. The new corporate enterprises relied on layers of salaried managers to coordinate the different aspects of the production and distribution of goods and services, such as amassing supplies, scheduling priorities and assignments, and meshing different kinds of labor.[35] Separate departments were set up to take care of different functions, each with its own management team. These large-scale organizations also required sizable accounting and clerical staffs to keep track of production, maintain records of costs, payrolls, materials, finished products, sales, and credit and, above all, to calculate profit and loss. The proliferation of consumer goods in turn fueled expansion in wholesale and retail sectors, expanding employment for counter clerks, cashiers, bookkeepers, account clerks, and other white-collar workers.

The ranks of management and supervisors were reserved exclusively for men. The salaries of higher managers afforded them an affluent lifestyle: well-furnished homes overseen by wives who had time for leisure pursuits because they could hire servants to assist them in household tasks. Middle managerial, administrative, and supervisory positions commanded monthly salaries that were sufficient to fulfill the male breadwinner ideal so that wives could remain at home. Clerical and retail sales jobs, although viewed as "respectable" white-collar positions, offered more modest salaries that might support a family, provided wives practiced frugality.

Ironically, during the height of the male wage-earner ideal, employment opportunities for women in clerical, secretarial, and sales jobs also grew. By 1929, over half of all clerical workers were women. Teaching, especially in public elementary schools, also became overwhelmingly female. Still, until the mid-twentieth century women usually left the labor force when they married or had children. Thus, the female white-collar and teaching sector was largely made up of young single women or married women without children or whose children were grown. In 1900 only 6 percent of white married women were counted as gainfully employed outside the home, a figure that rose to only 10 percent by 1930. As late as 1950, only 11.9 percent of women with children under age 6 were in the labor force.[36]

The emergence of the breadwinner ideal brought into being a complementary ideal, that of the "housewife." Although the term had been used earlier to describe women in family units where they performed productive and/or reproductive services, it now also came to refer to a

married woman who did not engage in productive (as opposed to reproductive) labor and who was economically dependent.[37] This change in
conception was codified by government in the way it categorized wom-
en's unpaid labor in the home. Nancy Folbre tracked changes in U.S.
Census classification of women's domestic labor over the course of the
nineteenth century. She notes, "In 1800, women whose work consisted
largely of caring for their families were considered productive workers.
By 1900, they had been formally relegated to the Census category of
"dependents," a category that included infants, young children, the sick,
and the elderly."[38] Christine Bose notes that between 1870 and 1930, U.S.
Census enumerators employed a double standard for assessing men's and
women's "gainful employment." Men were counted as gainfully employed
if they worked on family farms or family businesses, whereas women
similarly employed were not so counted. In general home-based labor
and labor that did not yield wages, as was the case for keeping boarders,
for example, was not counted. In this way, the Census reified dual
spheres ideology by severely undercounting women's labor and economic
contributions.[39]

Among middle-class families, the increasing range of consumer goods
contributed to a growing emphasis on housewives' consumption and
leisure activities. Larger and more elaborately furnished homes and
higher standards of cleanliness enlarged the volume of housework required to maintain a middle-class household. Mothering became more
central and labor intensive. Declines in infant mortality and birthrates
that started around 1800 continued throughout the nineteenth century.
Families had fewer children, so that each child came to be seen as having individual needs. In middle-class families, children no longer contributed labor and spent more years in school. Childhood came to be a
period of extended dependency during which children required protection and attentive care from a mother.[40]

Craft workers, who had some leverage, continued to fight for a living
wage. However, Lawrence Glickman argues that, unlike their antebellum counterparts, they no longer condemned the system of wage labor
itself but rather the inadequacy of the wages they received. Glickman
describes the shift as that from a producerist ethic to a consumerist
ethic: spokesmen for workingmen no longer appealed to the tenets of
productive republicanism but rather to the right to participate as equals
in the consumer market. Increasingly, a living wage was seen as en-

abling men and their families to enjoy an "American Standard of Living." This living standard included not only consumer goods but also an idealized family form with clearly differentiated gender roles.

Thus, nineteenth- and early twentieth-century labor leaders, such as Samuel Gompers, the president of the American Federation of Labor, fought to exclude women from skilled trades and supported lower wages for women on the grounds that they were only supplementing family income. The American standard of living was also racialized in that white working men saw black and other racial minority men as undermining the standard by being "willing" to work for less than white men. Some white leaders even claimed that blacks, Mexicans, and Chinese could sustain themselves at a lower standard, living in hovels and eating beans instead of meat, for example. Importantly for labor rights, the American Federation of Labor joined with employers in opposing minimum wage legislation on the grounds that such laws interfered with male unionists' ability to negotiate a living wage.

The opposition of the most visible and vocal element of organized labor to state protection contributed to the vulnerability of the vast majority of wageworkers, who were not organized.[41] Despite the supposed revolution in labor-saving technology, the corporate-dominated industrial economy relied heavily on the muscle power of so-called common laborers to perform the heavy physical labor required in mining, construction, and infrastructure building. Eugene Debs noted the importance of the common laborers, pointing out that "they perform the initial work in all enterprises."[42]

The actual numbers of common laborers is difficult to establish because the U.S. Census aggregated data by industries, often without specification of jobs. However, Alba Edwards, director of the 1910 U.S. Census, concluded that 32 percent of all male employees, nearly 10 million, deserved to be counted as common laborers.[43] Immigrant men from Europe, Asia, and Latin America and African American rural youth were particularly concentrated in common laborer jobs. Average daily wages were comparable to those of manufacturing jobs as a whole and higher than those paid in unskilled factory work; however, common laborer jobs tended to be seasonal and temporary, requiring workers to constantly search for employment and to move from job site to job site.[44]

For these workers, the ideal of the home as a domestic haven from economic striving was elusive. Women continued to engage in subsistence activity not only in rural and suburban areas but also in towns and cities. An 1890 study of 2,500 families in coal, iron, and steel regions found that nearly half raised poultry, livestock, and/or vegetable gardens in the grounds around their homes.[45] In that same period, families in Brooklyn and Manhattan north of midtown still engaged in small-scale agriculture. Given men's long hours in industrial or commercial employment, care of gardens and livestock fell mostly on women. Other urban women earned extra income at home by taking in boarders or renting rooms.[46] In some New York City immigrant tenements, apartments were turned into workshops as entire families engaged in various forms of industrial home work such as rolling cigars, sewing garments, and making hats for manufacturers. The labor of children remained important for the working class family economy, which relied on them to perform housework, take care of younger siblings, and help out with industrial outwork.[47] Thus, as in the preindustrial household, caring and income earning might take place alongside one another, and the home was not protected from the market or market values.

Still other families relied on multiple wage earners, with some combination of father, mother, other adults, and older children going out to work. Laurence Glasco found that working-class families typically enjoyed their greatest prosperity during the period when children were old enough to work but had not yet married.[48] There were also ethnic and racial differences in attitudes toward mothers' and children's employment. For example, Elizabeth Pleck found that in late nineteenth-century Philadelphia, among Italian families, mothers stayed home and sent children to work, whereas among black households mothers took jobs and tried to keep their children in school.[49] Similarly, S. J. Kleinberg found urban African American mothers engaged in much higher levels of wage work than white women in the period from 1880 to 1920, "using their own labor to delay their children's entry into the labor force."[50] Because many working-class women were not able to live up to the ideal of attentive full-time motherhood, working-class women were seen as inferior and insufficiently spiritual and uplifting caregivers.

Compared to the lack of respect for working-class and black women's domestic lives, the private household caring of middle-class and elite women was valorized and privileged. Yet, there was a fundamental contradiction between the spiritual qualities attributed to the ideal wife/mother and the heavy physical labor that was involved in caring. Keeping a house clean before the era of labor-saving devices required lots of elbow grease, scrubbing and sweeping floors and beating dusty rugs on an outside line. Cooking on iron stoves involved considerable advance preparation: fetching wood or coal, placing it in the fire compartment and lighting it, waiting for the oven and stovetop to be heated, and adding wood periodically to keep both at the right temperature. Laundering clothing and linen was a particularly arduous enterprise that took an entire day. Water had to be heated, items had to be scrubbed by hand, rinsed, wrung out, starched, and hung out to dry. Nursing sick children or elderly parents undoubtedly had its spiritual aspects, but it also entailed tending sores and wounds, cleaning up messes, changing bedding, and lifting invalids.[51]

This contradiction could be resolved if the menial physical labor could be separated from the spiritual and supervisory responsibilities and assigned to less privileged women. Moreover, affluent women and families were viewed as "needing" servants to create a home that reached the expected standard of cleanliness, order, and beauty. Elite women had always employed servants, but in the latter part of the nineteenth century, women of the middling classes also came to rely on paid household helpers. In major U.S. cities, the 1880 Census counted more than 15 servants per 100 families.[52] Who were these women who filled the ranks of cooks, maids, child nurses, housekeepers, and laundresses? In order to address this question, we now turn to the second historical thread, that of forced labor regimes.

Coercive Labor Regimes through the Early Republic

As settler colonies with relatively sparse populations, the economies of pre-Revolutionary America relied on bound workers to fill the need for labor. In the decades leading up to the American Revolution, three-quarters of new migrants were unfree workers: slaves, indentured servants, and convicts.[53]

African chattel slavery and white indentured servitude were both planted on American soil by the first English settlers. The initial group of bound Africans and indentured servants arrived in the American colonies in the early 1600s. The terms of their bondage at first were not clearly differentiated from one another. The two groups performed a similarly wide array of manual and skilled labor and often worked and lived alongside one another, leading in some cases to mixed unions. Slaves and servants were also subject to comparable treatment; they could be whipped for transgressions, arrested and sentenced to extended service for running away or violating the terms of their indenture, and sold or willed as property by their masters. The main difference—a monumental one—was that whereas indenture was for a fixed term, slavery was lifelong.[54]

Over the course of the seventeenth century, the status of slaves as hereditary chattel was regularized and differentiated from that of indentured servants.[55] Southern slave owners were motivated to regularize slave status in order to ensure there would be a permanent labor force for the expanding tobacco culture in the Chesapeake and upper South regions and for rice cultivation in the lower South. For example, Virginia decreed that the status of offspring followed the condition of the mother, so that children born of slave women were slaves. Slavery became clearly racialized, limited to blacks and Native Americans.[56] In contrast to white indenture, which declined after the American Revolution, black slavery continued to increase along with the expansion of southern agrarian and plantation economies.[57]

A growing movement against the Atlantic slave trade in Britain and the United States led the United States to ban the importation of slaves in 1808. However, by that time, slave owners could count on natural increase to replenish and even expand the population of slaves. The ban on importation did have some side effects: women increased as a proportion of the slave population, and they became more valuable because of their ability to enrich owners by producing additional slaves.[58]

Regarding gender divisions of labor, both bondsmen and bondswomen were forced into fieldwork and other hard outdoor labor. However, a significant proportion of women and children were assigned to household tasks, the dirty, heavy work of cleaning, laundering, and cooking as well as the nurturing work of nursing and caring for infants and children and tending to sick and disabled family members. Maternity did not excuse slave women from fieldwork or household labor. Although their ability to bear children was valued, the mothering of their own children and caring for kin was not. Those who spent long hours caring for the master's children and household had little time and energy for caring for their own; they also had no say about their children being drafted into labor at an early age. Older slave women, who were past their prime for fieldwork, might be assigned to watch all of the infants and young children, and elderly enslaved women known as "nurses" used their knowledge of herbs to treat sick and injured slaves.[59]

In the North, only Vermont and Massachusetts abolished slavery outright shortly after the end of the Revolution.[60] Additionally, the Northwest Ordinance of 1787 banned slavery in the territory that eventually became the states of Ohio, Indiana, Illinois, Michigan, and Wisconsin. However, most other northern states, including Pennsylvania, Connecticut, Rhode Island, New York, and New Jersey passed "gradual abolition" laws. Solicitous of owners' property rights, the legislatures in these states chose not to free any living slaves but limited the period of servitude of those born after the date the laws were passed. For example, under Connecticut's law, children born to slave parents after 1784 were released from servitude when they reached age 25.[61] These gradual abolition states later eliminated slavery, but the last, Connecticut and New Jersey, did not do so until the late 1840s.[62] In short, although the number of slaves had declined, legally sanctioned slavery survived in the north until 14 years before the Civil War.

Slave women in the North engaged in domestic service, cleaning, and laundering not only in their owners' households, but also in their workshops, taverns, boarding houses, and other public establishments. As noted earlier, scholars have documented the increase in white women (usually widows) running service establishments such as boarding houses and taverns in the late eighteenth and early nineteenth centuries. These women relied on the labor of other women, including slaves, to provide the domestic services, such as laundering and cleaning, that boarders and customers required.[63]

White indentured servants predominated among European immigrants throughout the colonial period. In the seventeenth century nearly 100,000 indentured servants entered compared to only two-thirds that number of free immigrants. In the subsequent three-quarters of a century (1700–1775), over 100,000 more indentured persons immigrated to the 13 colonies, although now outnumbered by an estimated 151,600 free immigrants; during this same period 278,400 slaves arrived. Among indentured immigrants, the proportion of English declined, but they were replaced by non-English-speaking servants, primarily Irish and German immigrants. German servants predominated among those headed for Philadelphia, where they arrived as "redemptioners." Under this system, before embarking, immigrants signed contracts stating how much time they had to get in touch with relatives, friends, or fellow villagers to redeem the cost of their fares. If they failed, they were auctioned off as indentured servants.[64]

Aaron S. Fogleman's careful analysis of existing records indicates that most early indentured immigrants voluntarily entered into indentures, temporarily forfeiting their freedom in exchange for passage, shelter, and sustenance. However, others entered indenture under less auspicious circumstances, as political exiles or debtors. Fogleman notes that at least in the seventeenth century, "The terms of service were longer in America, and the labor was generally more arduous, but the incentives via freedom dues were greater than in Britain. . . . Until about 1660 the chances were high that a young man who completed an indenture in the Chesapeake could achieve a comfortable position in society." But, by the mid-eighteenth century, living and working conditions had worsened, and opportunities for acquiring land had declined, so that it became difficult for freed servants to succeed. In letters to relatives, indentured servants described their conditions as miserable and advised others to "avoid indentured servitude if at all possible."[65]

Women initially constituted a small minority of indentured servants, but by the latter half of the eighteenth century, they constituted a larger share, suggesting an increasing demand for domestic servants.[66] According to Sharon Salinger in her study of indentured servants in Philadelphia:

> The work pace for female servants was similarly difficult and varied (as that of male servants). Domestic servants were accountable for a wide range of chores, from cooking and housework to carding and spinning, washing and "doing up the linen." Domestic tasks were endless, often disagreeable, and occasionally dangerous. Servants were required to be available twenty-four hours per day. Child care took up much of the time, and servants acted as wet nurses, as well as baby nurses, and tended children. . . . Domestic servants were called upon by their masters for the slightest excuse—a barking dog or a scary noise. They were also to be on hand for more serious matters in case of illness or when a fire alarm sounded.[67]

At least one servant had to rise before the family to stoke the fire and prepare hot beverages. To ensure their availability at night, some female servants slept on mats at the foot of their mistresses' bed.[68] Female servants were also vulnerable to sexual abuse and could be punished for getting pregnant by being whipped and having their terms extended. Mostly untrained in any but domestic tasks, many female servants faced bleak futures after completing their indentures. Records of the Philadelphia Guardians of the Poor reveal a higher proportion of former female servants were poor and in need of public aid compared to former male servants.[69]

A subtype of indentured servitude, convict labor, arose in the eighteenth century. This group was mostly made up of English, Scottish, and Irish criminals and political prisoners. During this period English prisons were overflowing with poor people, many convicted for petty theft and given the choice of hanging or transportation. From 1718, when Parliament passed the Transportation Act, until 1775, some 60,000 convicts dubbed "The King's Passengers" were transported in chains to America and auctioned off, still in chains, as indentured servants. They served primarily in Virginia and Maryland to fill labor needs in rice and tobacco agriculture. Indentured convicts served longer periods than voluntary indentured servants, typically for seven or fourteen years depending on the severity of the sentence. Like the terms of other indentured servants, the duration of convicts' servitude could be extended for violating the conditions of indenture. For example, servants who ran away and were recaptured had to serve anywhere from double to five times the amount of time that they were gone.[70]

The Revolutionary War decisively ended convict indenture because England could no longer use America as an outlet for its prisoners. After the Revolution, Parliament restarted the expulsion of convicts, redirecting them to a new British colony, Australia. The Revolution also disrupted the immigration of voluntary English indentured servants. However, the trade revived in the 1780s and 1790s, relying more heavily on German and Irish servants. The indenture system survived into the first two decades of the nineteenth century, although with diminishing numbers.[71]

Apprenticeships constituted the final major category of indentured labor. In a production system based on craft skills, apprenticing with a master craftsman was the major route to acquiring a trade. Well-to-do parents might pay to place their sons with merchants, lawyers, or other professionals to learn a profession. Middling parents placed their children in craft apprenticeships, which involved living and boarding with their masters and assisting them. Because of the boarding provision, some parents apprenticed their children to save themselves the cost of their upkeep, whereas still other parents indentured their children to settle debts. Additionally, pauper children and orphans were involuntarily placed in long-term apprenticeships by almshouses and orphan homes.[72] Apprenticeship contracts commonly required masters to provide food, clothing, shelter, as well as education, training, and "freedom dues" of clothes, tools, or money when the apprentice completed the period of indenture. In turn, the contracts enjoined apprentices to serve "faithfully and obediently" and to forswear prohibited behavior, such as gambling and fornication. Parents or town authorities transferred legal authority over children to the master for a substantial portion of their youth. This meant that masters also owned the apprentices' labor and any products and profit resulting from that labor. As in the case of indentured servants, boy apprentices received training that prepared them to become independent workers, whereas girl apprentices were assigned to learn "housewifery" under the supervision of mistresses and thus did not acquire an independent trade.[73]

The decline and eventual abolition of child apprenticeships and adult indentured servitude came about through a combination of economic and ideological factors. In the closing decades of the eighteenth century, economic downturns following the French and Indian Wars and disruptions in the flow of trade following the Revolution caused many small crafts operations, shops, and farms to fail. Concomitantly, opportunities for men to establish themselves as independent artisans and freeholders shrank. For the first time, the supply of "free labor" began to exceed demand, and wages of workers fell. In these circumstances, in some respects free workers became more attractive than bound workers. Unlike slaves or indentured servants, hired workers did not require employers to take on long-term obligations. Because they could be dismissed quickly, hired workers offered the employer greater flexibility in the face of economic uncertainty.[74]

The preference for waged labor was also promoted by democratic ideals fomented by the Revolution. White apprentices began running away more frequently and demanding journeymen's wages. Journeymen and mechanics formed associations and asserted their right to suffrage and other rights of citizenship based on ownership of their own labor. As noted earlier in this chapter, servitude had come to be seen as incongruent with (white) American manhood. By 1820, when white indentured servitude was legally banned, the practice had almost disappeared on its own.[75]

From the Civil War to the Early Twentieth Century

The Civil War and the passage of the Thirteenth, Fourteenth, and Fifteenth Amendments to the U.S. Constitution formally ended both slavery and indentured servitude. For a brief period during federal Reconstruction, many freed blacks enjoyed rights formerly denied them, including education, male suffrage, and the right of adults to contract their own labor. However, they were never given "freedom dues" of land and supplies as had been commonly granted to white indentured servants. When Reconstruction ended in the late 1870s, the vast majority of freedmen and women were bereft of the material resources that would have allowed them to become independent farmers, shopkeepers, and artisans.[76]

White southerners quickly took back political control. With the cooperation of an increasingly indifferent northern public, they succeeded in rewriting the history of slavery and Reconstruction to naturalize white supremacy. Wielding the banner of states' rights, southern Democrats formed a powerful bloc in the U.S. Congress to protect white southern interests and ward off any federal interference with white rule. Southern legislatures, public officials, and courts systematically disenfranchised blacks, mandated segregation in public facilities and work sites, and conspired with land owners and employers to reestablish forced labor regimes as close to slavery as possible. These included signing freedmen to "voluntary" labor contracts that differed little from indentured servitude. Black subordination was also buttressed by extralegal means, including terror and violence.[77]

After a brief period of using work gangs as they had under slavery, plantation owners turned to tenancy arrangements, the most common of which was "going on halves." Owners allotted small plots to individual sharecroppers and provided rations, seeds, fertilizer, and other supplies on credit in exchange for half the crop. Propertyless tenants had little choice but to borrow for supplies at exorbitant rates of interest—up to 25 percent—secured by a lien on the year's crop. These arrangements effectively tied sharecroppers down for the season and also impelled wives and children to work in the fields to maximize yields. Contracts were renegotiated at the end of the season when all debts had been settled. In a good year, a sharecropper might clear a few hundred dollars, but in a bad year, he might wind up still in debt. When the landlord was also the creditor, the system constituted debt peonage.[78]

Although agriculture was the main industry that imposed peonage, it was by no means the only one. Railroads, mines, sawmills, turpentine extractors, and construction firms relied heavily on debt bondage and penal contracts. For example, in the turpentine industry, workers were housed in compounds surrounded by barbed wire and watched over by armed guards. Workers were forced to buy necessities from company commissaries on credit. Workers who attempted to quit while owing money to the employer could be charged with fraudulently procuring money and sentenced to a choice of a long prison sentence or compulsory labor.[79]

Southern legislatures used criminal laws to compel labor. For example, to prevent workers from leaving when they wanted to, legislatures passed "enticement laws" that made it a crime to hire anyone employed by or under contract to another.

Even more widespread were vagrancy statutes. Under these laws, local law enforcement officers could apprehend "idlers" and impose fines they could not pay. Local officials would then hire the "idlers" out to work off their fines, usually as servants or common laborers, in road construction, land reclamation, fieldwork, or digging mines. Black women were included among those subject to arrest for vagrancy. Unlike their white counterparts, married black women supported by husbands were assumed to be idle if not working for wages. In times of shortage of domestic servants, black women were particularly likely to be targeted for arrest.[80]

Southern states also passed laws making petty crimes into felonies that entailed long sentences. Under Mississippi's 1876 "Pig Law," the theft of a farm animal or property worth more than $10 was defined as grand larceny, punishable by no less than 5 years in prison. Thousands of mostly black poor were arrested, summarily convicted, and leased out to state and private contractors. From the 1870s to the 1920s (when Alabama was the last state to abolish convict leasing), prisoners cleared land and built levees in Mississippi, bore tunnels and laid railroad tracks in Tennessee and South Carolina, mined coal in Alabama's Birmingham coal district, and collected turpentine in Florida swampland to supply the U.S. Navy. By 1890 Alabama was running what amounted to a state-operated slave market for its prisoners: black men aged 12 and older were sorted into four grades at different prices for work in mines; black women, children, and "cripples" were sent to lumber camps and farms. Meanwhile white male criminals remained in penitentiaries and jails, and white female and juvenile offenders were sent to special facilities.[81]

In the industrial North and Midwest de facto, rather than de jure means were employed to keep African Americans in a state of subjugation. Black men were shut out of white-collar positions, skilled trades, and mechanized jobs, regardless of their qualifications. Black men worked as common laborers on construction sites, in rail yards, and in industrial plants and as servants and janitors in service establishments.[82] Because of strict segregation of occupations, black men were occasionally able to monopolize particular jobs. Of the service jobs reserved for black men, that of Pullman porter on trains was the most visible and respected in the African American community.[83] Black women were shut out of typical female occupations such as retail sales, clerical jobs, and light assembly work, and the majority were concentrated in various branches of domestic work in private homes and service enterprises such as commercial laundries.[84]

In short, black men and women were overwhelmingly stuck in low-paid, dead-end jobs and denied any chance of promotion to skilled or supervisory positions. The jobs that many black men and women held were insecure and seasonal as well as low paid, so they could not accumulate resources and had no economic cushion to fall back on. Under those circumstances, they had to take whatever job was offered and to endure horrendous conditions, or face starvation.

In parts of the West and Southwest, where local economies were based on primary industries (agriculture, extraction, and infrastructure development) and the labor force was heavily made up of workers of color (Indians, Mexicans, and Asians), peonage also thrived. In New Mexico, formerly independent sheep owners were forced into "share sheeping" in the 1880s after getting enmeshed in credit extended by Anglo merchants. Unable to pay their loans, herders had their sheep seized and leased back to them by creditors.[85] In Texas cotton agriculture,

Mexican tenant farmers were subject to debt bondage similar to that experienced by southern black sharecroppers.[86] In Colorado, coal mining companies paid workers in scrip that could be redeemed in full only at the company store, effectively tying them down by making their earnings worthless outside of the camp.[87]

And, in contravention of U.S. laws against contract labor, railroad companies and agribusinesses procured gang labor through labor agents who recruited workers not only within the region but also in Mexico. Agents typically withheld 25 percent of the workers' wages until the end of the season or contractual period and also deducted the cost of food and transportation. One observer reported that labor agents in Texas transported Mexican workers in chains to the worksite, where they were watched over by guards.[88] In nineteenth-century California many Chinese workers, including those who did the dangerous job of igniting explosives to bore tunnels and the arduous job of laying track, were bound laborers. They had arrived under the "credit ticket system," having signed contracts with intermediaries who hired them out to pay off the cost of their passage with interest, much as white indentured servants had done in the colonial period.[89]

Coercion was not limited to black workers and other workers of color. Under existing contract law, employers could sign workers to contracts with pay not forthcoming until the contractual period was complete. If the worker worked 10 months on a 12-month contract and left, he forfeited all wages. While waiting for wages, the worker might live on credit extended by the employer. Any debt had to be paid in full immediately upon quitting or the worker would be subject to criminal prosecution for fraud. In these cases, employers used "voluntary" labor contracts entered into by theoretically free and equal parties to immobilize workers and compel labor.[90]

Robert J. Steinfeld investigated the contradiction between theoretical freedom and substantive bondage to broaden the definition of labor coercion. Steinfeld defines coercion as any circumstance in which one can only choose between two evils. Labor coercion occurs when performing disagreeable labor is preferable to an even more disagreeable alternative. How disagreeable does the alternative have to be for it to be considered worse than illegitimate servitude? In the nineteenth century, U.S. courts usually drew a line between non-pecuniary and pecuniary sanctions, defining only non-pecuniary sanctions as impermissible compulsion. For example, imprisonment for non-performance was deemed to constitute servitude, whereas forfeiture of accumulated wages if a worker left before the end of a contractual period was not viewed as servitude.

Not until the late nineteenth century did these practices begin to be challenged. Starting in 1879, state legislatures, in response to pressure from organized labor, began to pass laws that required regular payment of wages, usually monthly or biweekly. Some states also passed legislation that required employers to pay in cash or scrip redeemable in cash instead of scrip redeemable only in company stores, as well as laws that required employers to pay back wages for days worked if the worker left before the end of a pay period. Yet, as late as 1935, one-third of states, presumably those with weak labor movements, still had no wage laws on their books.[91]

Intersections of Home and Coerced Labor

We have seen that marketization and industrialization fundamentally transformed the household economy by making it increasingly reliant on earnings from wage labor. Although women continued to engage in subsistence activity, their primary responsibilities were defined as homemaking, child care, and consumption. The content of these activities might vary by economic class (creating and displaying a desired lifestyle for middle-class families, and carefully managing purchases to make ends meet for working-class and poor families), but they were similarly viewed as non-economic in nature. Importantly, from an ideological perspective, as embodied in the law and in everyday understandings, these unpaid responsibilities were stripped of economic significance and instead viewed as moral and spiritual vocations. In contrast to men's paid labor, women's unpaid caring was simultaneously priceless and worthless—that is, not monetized.

Further, unpaid care work came to be equated with dependence. From the early nineteenth century on, working and earning were the bases for white men to claim independence. The figure of the independent male wage earner brought into being the contrasting figure of the dependent housewife. Housewives were treated as, and usually thought of themselves as, economic dependents of a male breadwinner. The breadwinner ideal for men meant that even if wives were employed, their earnings were seen as supplementing that of the primary family earner.

For middle-class women, the changes carried contradictory implications, between the elevation of their caring labor in spiritual, moral, and altruistic terms on the one hand and the devaluation of that same labor in economic and political terms on the other. An economic system that counted only monetized labor and a political system that made earning the basis for entitlements of citizenship effectively excluded and rendered invisible unpaid caring. A second set of contradictions arose from the valorization of spiritual labor as an expression of superior morality and the denigration of bodily labor as an expression of baseness. Caring labor involved both types of work; yet it was only the supervisory and nurturing aspects that were valued, while the heavy physical parts of caring (often involving dirty work) were devalued. But these contradictions could be bridged if the two aspects of caring could be assigned to different groups of women.

This is where the lives of privileged women intersected with poor women and women of color, who were members of groups subjected to coercive labor regimes. Historically, caring labor in the homes of more privileged classes was split between wives, mothers, and daughters on the one hand and servants drawn from the ranks of the less-privileged classes on the other. In the United States, the less-privileged classes included slaves, indentured servants, immigrants, and subordinated minorities who were locked into coercive labor regimes.

An integral aspect of systems of labor coercion, whether formal slavery, indenture, debt bondage, convict leasing, or other forms of compulsion, was appropriation of not only men's and women's productive labor but also women's reproductive labor—that is, caring labor. Whereas men in subordinated groups were commonly compelled to perform hard physical labor in agriculture, construction, and mining, women and girls were directed into domestic service, where they performed caring labor for their social superiors.

Compulsion to provide care for others could take many forms, similar to those used to compel other kinds of labor. These ranged from labor market segregation and discrimination that closed off other ways of earning a living to welfare laws that denied black and Mexican single mothers benefits so that they would be forced to take on domestic employment. This use of welfare regulations to impel single mothers into the labor force, even in the absence of job training and a living wage, is a strategy that has been periodically deployed up to the present day.

In situations where one industry or employer dominated an area, the compulsion might be highly personal, as in the case of plantation managers and overseers "requesting" that workers send their daughters or wives to work in their homes. The not so subtle threat—the loss of the primary earner's job—was well understood by workers and their families. In other cases, as noted previously, criminal law was deployed, as in the case of vagrancy laws that allowed local officials to sentence black women who were not employed to jobs as domestic servants. The threat in these cases was incarceration, which might also entail vulnerability to rape and other violence. This dire situation fits precisely Steinfeld's definition of coercion as having only two disagreeable options from which to choose. In this case, blacks were forced to choose between performing hard, unpleasant work or suffering a severe penalty (e.g., jail or starvation).

A second very important, but often neglected corollary feature was the negative impact of coercive labor regimes on the ability of workers and their families to receive care from and provide care for their own kin. The middle-class ideal was that families took care of their own and that women as wives and mothers bore primary responsibility for providing care. Middle-class women were thus prevailed upon to devote more or less full time to care work. However, the labor system, which was coercive for men and women of color specifically and for working-class and poor men and women generally, hampered families' efforts to care for their own and drew mothers' and wives' labor away from focused caring for their own families.

To add insult to injury, because they could not live up to the ideal of full-time motherhood, poor women of color were seen as deficient mothers and caregivers. These "deficiencies" were often cited as the cause of a lack of moral character among the poor, and of deprivations suffered by their children. Dominant ideology thus turned attention away from economic inequality and focused it on individual and familial deficiencies and dysfunctions.

Women of color offered alternative perspectives on motherhood and caregiving. Employed African American mothers did not see themselves as deficient mothers just because they worked outside the home. African American mothers saw economic provision as part of being a good mother. In fact, as mentioned previously about different responses to the need for income among working-class families, African American mothers were more likely to work outside the home themselves rather than send children out to work as white working-class families did. They preferred to keep their children in school as long as possible, probably to increase their children's chances at a better life.

Changes in Home Caregiving for the Ill and Disabled

Home nursing was one of the most arduous responsibilities that white women and women of color carried prior to the mid-twentieth century. In her study of caregiving in the nineteenth century, Emily Abel found that free women provided nursing not only for immediate family members but also for a wide circle of kin and neighbors. Arrangements to relieve women of their responsibilities for care were scarce. Most nineteenth-century Americans never saw the inside of a hospital, and physicians were often too far away and their services too expensive for most households. Women caregivers thus provided the bulk of nursing care, preparing meals, cleaning up messes, sitting at bedsides, and administering home-made medicines, such as oil and turpentine and gum camphor. They relied on their own knowledge and skills, which they had learned from observing and assisting other caregivers. Abel notes: "Because infectious diseases were rampant, infants and children frequently required nursing care. Common killers included pneumonia, typhus, typhoid fever, diphtheria, scarlet fever, measles, whooping cough, dysentery, and tuberculosis. During epidemics, women moved continually from house to house in the community, exposing themselves and their own families to disease. Women also received frequent calls to lend assistance at deliveries." Because sickness often led to death, "care giving also had an important spiritual component. . . . Women sought to ensure that dying people were adequately penitent, 'sensible' of their sins, and prepared to face their death with equanimity." After a person's death a caregiver might assist with preparing and dressing the body and in making linings and pillows for the coffin.[92]

In letters and diaries white women expressed a strong sense of duty to provide care. Married women talked about their exhausting routines combining caring for the sick with their usual household work. Single daughters spoke about giving up education or jobs to care for a parent or other relative. Abel notes, "In her autobiography, Lucy Sprague Mitchell, a famous educator recalled that she had not questioned her family's expectation that she would nurse her parents and cousin. 'As a dutiful daughter, I simply did my job . . . I accepted the standards of the time that daughters belonged to their families.'" Even a high-status professional position did not excuse a daughter from her caring obligations. "Mary Holywell Everett was a successful New York physician when her sister became ill in 1876. A male colleague to whom she had written counseled her thus: 'Even at the risk of losing your practice entirely, duty commands you to remain by the side of your old mother and help her carry the burden.'"[93]

Within the community of slaves, caregiving was also women's work. Wilma Dunaway, in her study of slave families in the Appalachian region, found that

> self treatment was the primary medical strategy of the vast majority of mountain slaves. . . . Mothers tended their own families until the illness grew too complicated, then they called on one of their community healers. Elderly "root doctors" or "herb healers" handled community health care, and some old women too old for field work often cared for the sick. . . . The most expert slave healers were *conjurers* who were able to diagnose and treat complex conditions with herbal concoctions, charms, diets, and physical regimes. Combining African and Native American knowledge about indigenous plants, these healers used a variety of teas, poultices, and ointments derived from plants gathered from the woods or cultivated in garden parcels.[94]

However, slave caregivers were often not allowed to use their knowledge and skills but instead were directed to administer remedies provided by the slaveowner. Emily Abel notes, "Enslaved people complained that white medicine was less effective than African American treatments, had no power when diseases were caused by supernatural forces, and sometimes caused harm. One former slave reported that the calomel a white doctor administered 'would pretty nigh kill us.'" Also, slave women, unlike white women, were not allowed to give priority to their own family members and had to fight to care for their own. As a result, caregiving had to be done in the interstices of time around the work required by their owners. According to Abel, crowded habitation and the burden of field labor fostered collective approaches to caregiving, which in turn reinforced bonds of kinship and community. Despite the obstacles, "the caregiving work of enslaved women subverted the plantation regime in subtle ways. Women concealed children's illnesses, substituted herbal brews for calomel and quinine, bestowed loving care and compassion on family members whom owners viewed only as labor power, and strove to preserve communities in the face of a system that constantly threatened their survival."[95]

With the growth of formal health care systems in the late nineteenth and early twentieth centuries, family caregivers of all classes, races, and ethnicities lost much of their autonomy, and their traditional knowledge became devalued. Allopathic medicine, which claimed to be based on scientific methods, became dominant, and other types of medicine, such as homeopathy, were marginalized. In the early 1900s the American Medical Association (AMA) was reorganized into a confederation of state associations (which in turn were confederations of county associations), thus unifying physicians under one umbrella and making the AMA the authorized voice of the profession. At the urging of the AMA, the Carnegie Foundation conducted an investigation of medical schools. The resulting Flexner Report of 1910 recommended a drastic reduction in the number of medical schools and the standardization of medical training. During this same period, states and medical associations were implementing reforms in medical education and licensing requirements that were leading to consolidation of smaller medical schools and closure of marginal ones. Within five years the number of medical schools in the United States fell from 131 to 95, and the annual number of medical school graduates dropped from 5,440 to 3,536.[96]

Simultaneously, however, the number of hospitals increased. Whereas in 1873 there were 178 medical and mental hospitals in the United States, by 1923 there were 6,830. Thus instead of care at home, hospitalization became more common. The rise in hospitalization, combined with the drop in the number of physicians, created a demand for skilled nursing labor, leading in turn to the rise of nursing schools and the professionalization of nursing. Never achieving the power, prestige, or exclusivity of medicine, hospital nursing remained a heterogeneous field in terms of level and types of training and education. Nonetheless, nursing leaders claimed their nurses' superiority over untrained nurses by claiming specialized technical skills and abstract knowledge.[97]

The professionalization of medicine and nursing and the growth of hospitals led to the devaluing of informal family care. According to Abel, nineteenth-century physicians often valued personal relations as a way to relieve stress and as a source of knowledge. By the early twentieth century, physicians increasingly disparaged the emotional aspects of health care. In the opinion of many physicians, family caregivers tended to coddle patients and failed to impose regimens necessary to promote healing. Medical administrators advocated hospitalization for an increasing range of ailments, arguing that patients needed the order and discipline imposed by trained medical personnel. Meanwhile, "patients remaining at home were enjoined to place themselves under the control of credentialed nurses if at all possible." Wives and mothers continued to provide home nursing, but their work became less autonomous because it was ideally to be carried out under a physician's direction. Lay caregivers were warned not to rely on folk knowledge but to seek authoritative advice from physicians.[98]

3

The Movement to Reform Women's Caring

The late nineteenth century saw the rise of several overlapping social currents that converged to draw elite women into movements to reform society and to uplift less fortunate women. Social feminism, a movement grounded in a belief in inherent differences between the sexes and the existence of distinct male and female spheres, glorified women's domestic roles as mothers and "keepers of the home." Social feminists viewed women's domesticity as essential to maintaining the home and hetero-patriarchal family, which they considered to be the cornerstones of a moral and civilized society.

The social purity movement, a moral campaign dedicated to cleaning up society, began in the 1870s when former abolitionists organized to emancipate prostitutes, whom they referred to as "white slaves." The effort grew into a multifaceted movement with different branches mounting crusades against drinking, gambling, and venereal disease and in favor of sex education, moral education, and a strong American family. Christian, Nativist, and eugenic sentiments animated many of these crusades. A third current was Progressivism, a political movement that also sought to improve society but was wider in scope and more secular in approach. According to historian Nicole Rafter, "Idealistic and moralistic, Progressives proposed to make government responsive to an increasingly urban, industrial and ethnically mixed society."[1] Progressives believed in capitalism but abandoned the older notion that it was self-regulating. They looked to the state to play a critical role in reigning in the excesses of capitalism and protecting those who were weak or vulnerable and thus unable to fend for themselves in the market. The

Progressives also sought political means to advance democratic citizenship by raising the level of the citizenry through improved education, public health, and standards of living.[2]

Aspiring women reformers such as Florence Kelley, Lillian Wald, Julia Lathrop, and Edith Abbott drew on the tenets of social feminism to make the case that women's experiences as "keepers of the home" made them particularly well suited to play a similar role as moral guardians of society as a whole. They expanded women's caring mission to encompass the public arena, carving out a specifically gendered role for themselves in social purity and progressive reform. In accordance with the doctrine of separate spheres, elite women claimed their special province as uplifting less fortunate women, children, and families.

Elite women formed their own organizations dedicated to eradicating corrupting influences and also joined in progressive reform, concentrating on improving the situation of women, children, and families in the city. As individuals and as members of progressive groups, they lobbied state and local officials to pass legislation to protect women workers, to monitor hours and safety conditions in factories, to improve sanitation in tenement neighborhoods, and to establish standards for tenement housing. Following the example of Jane Addams's Hull House in Chicago, Progressive women established settlement houses that conducted surveys of living conditions and provided services in poor and working-class neighborhoods. During the 1910s former settlement house leaders took positions in state and federal agencies that were established to promote the well-being of children, mothers, and employed women. They also started new women's professions, such as social work, home economics, and home nursing, to carry out reform directly in the field.[3]

One particular subset of elite women's "public caring" activities was to remake non-elite women to fit elite concepts of women as keepers of the home. These reform projects aimed at "domesticating" girls and women deemed to be inadequately womanly by the standards of the dominant culture. Gender was a central organizing principle of these projects, not just because the agents and targets were women but also because the goal was to produce subjects who willingly undertook their gender-assigned duties and obligations.

Three women-led and women-targeting movements stood out in the period from the 1870s to the 1930s:

Assimilation programs for Native American girls that entailed removing them from their families and placing them in Indian boarding schools where they could be trained in Anglo-American domestic skills.

Reformatory programs for females convicted of morals offenses that involved incarcerating them in all-female institutions run by women where they could be rehabilitated to become working class mothers and domestic servants.

Americanization programs for immigrant mothers that sought to reform their housekeeping, cooking, and child care practices to accord with Anglo-American norms.

Each of these projects was part of a larger reform movement that included both men and women, to assimilate Indians, to reform and rehabilitate prisoners, and to "Americanize" immigrants. Each of the larger movements has been studied by scholars but in isolation rather than in relation to the others. Moreover, the movements have not been analyzed specifically in terms of how they targeted women's caring behavior. By bringing the three projects under the common analytic framework of caring labor, we can shed light on underlying ideologies and practices that link them. The claim is not that reforming "other women's" caring was the sole or primary objective of the larger movements but that it constituted a significant component of each intervention and that, taken together, they demonstrate how women's and subordinates' obligation to care was recodified during a critical period in American history when women's citizenship was being expanded.

"Acculturating" Native Americans

In the latter half of the nineteenth century, U.S. government policy toward Native Americans became focused on assimilation or, as it was often dubbed, "Americanization."[4] The aim of the assimilation policy was to phase out treaty rights and other special statuses of Native Americans, and thereby to absorb them into the dominant society.

The twin prongs of Indian assimilation policy were land allotment and education. Allotment would privatize tribal lands into individual plots assigned to families and individuals. By allotting larger holdings to heads of households, the program would encourage the formation of nuclear households. Proponents of allotment believed that owning and working individual plots would transform Indian men into citizen farmers and Indian women into farm wives.[5] Education would complement allotment by preparing Indians for their new productive roles in U.S. society. Special schools for Indians would be set up to inculcate them in Christianity, English, vocational skills, and self-discipline. Importantly, and not emphasized in previous scholarship, assimilation policy was intended to instill a sense of gender-appropriate duties and obligations: Indian men would learn to fulfill their responsibilities as heads of households by engaging in productive economic activity, and Indian women would learn to fulfill their duties as wives by engaging in caring activities within the home.[6]

Assimilation policy was carried out through the combined efforts of federal agencies and private religious and reform organizations. Government officials and agents at the Bureau of Indian Affairs (BIA) supported assimilation and acculturation as the best way to solve the "Indian problem" and to satisfy the white hunger for land by opening up "surplus" Indian country to white settlement. White "Friends of Indians" championed allotment, arguing that it would create some security for Indians by protecting some of their land from white encroachment. As a spokesman for the Indian Rights Association opined, "The friends of the new law think half a loaf better than no bread, even for Indians."[7]

Perhaps because of the long history of white–Indian conflict and Indian resistance, white men in the BIA were primarily concerned with civilizing Indian men. However, they came to agree that Americanizing Indian women was necessary in order to accomplish this primary task. For them the main rationale for uplifting Indian women was to motivate Indian men to strive. Similar to the placement of blame on strong black women for the plight of black men during the 1960s debates about the black family and poverty, the white men of the BIA a century earlier blamed Indian women for the "backwardness" of Indian men. In their view, the fact that Indian women carried out physical labor and were ignorant of "modern" housekeeping methods accounted for Indian men's laziness and disinterest in material progress. If Indian women could be educated to focus on the household and to desire better furnishings, Indian men would be impelled to work hard to acquire material goods.[8]

White women reformers were more likely to focus on the importance of reforming Indian women to achieve progress in the next generation. According to Merial A. Dorchester, a field supervisor in the Indian Schools,

> It is very clear to those most closely studying the "Indian problem" that the elevation of the women is, to a greater degree than many realize, the key to the situation. That the men are from 15 to 25 years in advance of the women is a no more freely admitted fact than that the children start from the plane of the mother rather than from that of the father. Therefore the great work of the present is to reach and lift the women and the home.[9]

Gender was a central organizing principle of assimilation programs. As noted previously, men and women would have to be trained to assume specific gender-appropriate duties and obligations. Education for Indian boys was aimed at training them in agriculture and trades, while education for Indian girls focused on domestic arts, housekeeping, and childcare. And the doctrine of separate spheres dictated that just as white men were the most appropriate teachers for Indian men, white women were viewed as uniquely qualified to reshape Indian womanhood in their own image.

In fact, elite and middle-class white women were actively involved in all phases of Indian reform, but with special focus on uplifting Indian women. White women leaders and members of the Women's National Indian Association circulated mass petitions to influence government policy in favor of land allotment and raised money and supplies to carry out private missionary and educational efforts. At a time when the federal government provided few resources for Indian education, these private fund-raising efforts constituted a significant source of material support. Other white women were employed as officials in the Office of the Commissioner of Indian Affairs in the 1890s and in its successor agency, the BIA, in the 1900s, where they helped to create and implement assimilation programs. One of the most influential of these women was Estelle Reel, who served as the Director of Indian Education from 1898 to 1910 during the peak years of Indian boarding schools. In addition to influencing and forming policy, white women constituted the majority of those who worked directly with Indian children and adult women as missionaries, teachers, school matrons, field matrons, and field nurses.[10]

White women's views of Indian women were shaped by eighteenth- and nineteenth-century colonial conceptions of indigenous societies as being backward and in need of uplift. Missionaries, colonial officials, and settlers wrote texts excoriating the "primitive" religious and marital practices of indigenous peoples. Furthermore, Euro-American commentators believed that their own idealized organization of gender represented the highest form of civilization. When they observed indigenous women doing heavy labor outdoors, they saw them not as strong and productive but as degraded and oppressed. Thus, one of the most common negative stereotypes of the Indian woman was as "squaw drudge."[11]

The drudge stereotype, widespread from the eighteenth century on, was shared by federal officials such as the Commissioner of Indian Affairs, who quoted an unnamed writer in his annual report of 1888: "His squaw was his slave. With no more affection than a coyote feels for its mate, he brought her to his wigwam that she might gratify the basest of his passions and minister to his wants. It was Starlight or Cooing Dove that brought the wood for his fire and the water for his drink, that plowed the field and sowed the maize." White women observers echoed this view. Frances S. Calfee, who served as a field matron for the Hualapais, wrote in 1896 that "the Hualapai women occupy an unenviable position, being counted little, if any, better than the dogs, and certainly not so valuable as the horses." Similarly, Mary Dissette, who worked for many years at the Zuni Pueblo, said that in Indian tribes, "the male is supreme and all that contributes to his comfort or pleasure is his by right of his male supremacy. The female is taught this from early childhood."[12]

Other negative views focused on Indian's women's defective caregiving, noting especially their "strange" infant care practices. A mid-nineteenth century observer, Catherine Haun, wrote: "The squaws carried their papooses in queer little canopied baskets suspended upon their backs by a band around their heads and across their foreheads. The infant was snugly bound, mummy-fashion with only its head free. It was here that I first saw a bit of remarkable maternal discipline, peculiar to most of the Indian tribes. The child cried whereupon the mother . . . stood it up against a tree and dashed water in the poor little creature's face." Half a century later, a missionary, a Miss Howard, reported: "I found a woman with a sick baby not yet three weeks old; of course it was strapped upon a board; and it was moaning with fever."[13]

From the white point of view, Indian women were also slovenly housekeepers. According to a federal official, even when moved into modern houses, Indian women took with them "the habits of out-of-door life—irregular meals, rarely washed cooking utensils and clothes, an assortment of dogs, a general distribution among corners and on the floors of bedding and personal belongings, and a readiness to consider the floor a not inconvenient substitute for bedsteads, tables, and chairs." The resulting "dirt, disease, and degradation" were deemed "the natural consequences" of Indian women's inadequate domestic skills.[14]

Allotment

The General Allotment Act of 1887 (the "Dawes Act") established the first government program for dividing reservation land into individual allotments. Instead of dividing up the total acreage of reservation land among individuals, the Act limited the size of allotments and gave different size allotments to individuals based on their family status. The largest allotments, 160 acres, were allotted to family heads, 80 acres for each single person over the age of 18, and 40 acres for orphans and any other single persons under age 18. A patent was to be issued for each allotment in the name of the allottee with the land held in trust by the government for 25 years, during which time the allottee could not sell the land or be taxed for it. At the end of the 25 years each allottee would be granted citizenship and granted the patent in fee. After the allotments were made to every member of the tribe, the government could negotiate with the tribe for purchase of the lands for the purpose of conveying the "surplus" lands to (white) settlers. In this way hundreds of thousands of acres of tribal lands were lost to white settlement.[15]

The rationale for the allotment program was explained by its sponsor, Senator Henry L. Dawes: "They have got as far as they can go, because they own their land in common. . . . There is no enterprise to make your home any better than that of your neighbors. There is no selfishness, which is at the bottom of civilization. Till this people will consent to give up their lands, and divide them among their citizens so that each can own the land he cultivates, they will not make much more progress."[16]

Education

The reformers' design for the education of Indian children consisted of two components, child removal and placement in boarding schools. For many proponents of assimilation, exposure and proximity to white Christian models were as important as direct tuition. They thus advocated for removing children from mothers' influence and care and educating them in boarding schools where the children would be taught by white women. Estelle Reel, Superintendent of Indian Schools, explained the need for removal: "the Indian child must be placed in school before the habits of barbarous life have become fixed, and there he must be kept until contact with our life has taught him to abandon his savage ways and walk in the path of Christian civilization." Reel strongly advocated for compulsory rather than voluntary school attendance: "If the Indian will not accept the opportunities for elevation and civilization so generously offered him," Reel asserted, "the strong hand of the law should be evoked and the pupil forced to receive an education whether his parents will it or not."[17]

As for the content of education, vocational training was emphasized with boys being prepared for farming and trades and girls for domestic activities. For Indian girls, the focus was on training them to create a "proper" American home, which meant inculcation in Christianity, cleanliness, and hygiene, the practice of economy (thriftiness), adoption of "American" childrearing practices, and domestic skills in sewing, cooking, home nursing, laundry, and cleaning. Because it was anticipated that Indians would make only a modest living, much emphasis was put on teaching Indian girls that they could create a cozy home with little expenditure.[18]

Superintendent Reel later opined: "Industrial training will make . . . the Indian girl more motherly. This is the kind of girl we want—the one who will exercise the greatest influence in moulding the character of the nation. . . . Thus will they become useful members of this great Republic, and if compulsory education is extended to all the tribes, there is little reason to doubt that the ultimate civilization of the race will result."[19]

White women participated in both removal and schooling; they were advocates for removing Indian children from their families as well as agents to help in the removal. As noted above, Estelle Reel was a prominent proponent of child removal. When the first boarding schools were being established, white women were often employed as recruiters to persuade Indian mothers to send their children away to school, offering the promise of a better life for them. For example, Alice Fletcher was hired to accompany U.S. Army captain Richard Henry Pratt to travel to reservations to recruit Indian children for the first boarding school program, which was established at the Hampton Institute in Virginia. In the boarding schools, white women constituted the majority of teachers and staff. White women also were employed as school matrons to maintain living quarters and to create a "homelike" situation within what was otherwise a military school environment.[20]

The Indian Boarding School System

The Hampton Institute, founded during Reconstruction by General Samuel C. Armstrong to educate recently freed blacks, enrolled a group of 18 Indians in 1878. The students had been part of a group of prisoners held by Captain Pratt at Fort Marion, Florida. Pratt had persuaded the government to educate 18 of the younger prisoners at Hampton. Both Armstrong and Pratt were pleased with the results and believed girls should be added to the program. In fact, Armstrong stipulated that Hampton would take Indian students only on the condition that there be an equal number of girls and boys. According to Armstrong "without educated women there is no civilization."[21]

Pratt, accompanied by his wife, traveled up the Missouri River to recruit 50 students. The Pratts had no problem enrolling boys but found that Indian mothers objected to having girls taken from home because they wanted to educate the girls themselves. Nonetheless, the Pratts succeeded in bringing nine girls to enroll the first year, and by 1880 there were 20 girls enrolled. Hampton developed a program for girls' education focusing on English and housekeeping skills that became the general model of boarding school training for Indian girls.[22]

Pratt had been concerned about racial mixing between blacks and Indians, and in 1879, he successfully petitioned the federal government to establish a separate Indian school at Carlisle, Pennsylvania. By 1880, 57 girls were enrolled at Carlisle.

As rapidly as possible the girls were placed in a system that put maximum emphasis on domestic chores. Academic learning clearly played a subordinate role. The girls spent no more than half a day in the classroom and devoted the rest of their time to domestic work. At Carlisle the first arrivals were instructed in "the manufacture and mending of garments, the use of the sewing machine, laundry work, cooking, and the routine of household duties pertaining to their sex."[23]

Pratt saw the education of native girls as supportive of the more important work of Americanizing native boys: "Of what avail is it, that the man be hardworking and industrious, providing by his labor food and clothing for his household, if the wife, unskilled in cookery, unused to the needle, with no habits of order or neatness, makes what might be a cheerful, happy home only a wretched abode of filth and squalor?" In some ways the girls' tasks were more complicated, for while an Indian boy need learn only one trade, an Indian girl "must learn to sew and to cook, to wash and iron, she must learn lessons of neatness, order, and economy, for without a practical knowledge of all these she cannot make a home."[24]

Three other important boarding schools, located closer to the tribes from which they drew students, were Chilocco, established in 1884 in Oklahoma; Haskell, established in 1884 in Lawrence, Kansas; and Phoenix Indian School, established in 1891 in Arizona. Phoenix's program for girls put even more emphasis on domestic training and less on classical subjects, such as art and history, than either Hampton or Carlisle. At Phoenix, female students performed all of the housework, including cooking, laundry, and cleaning, for the entire school. Elaborating on the industrial cottage system established at Hampton, "Phoenix operated a 'well-regulated household' run by nine girls under a matron's supervision. The 'family' (with no males present) cleaned and decorated the cottage, did the regular routine of cooking, washing, and sewing, and tended to the poultry and livestock in an effort 'to train them to the practical and social enjoyment of the higher life of a real home.'"[25]

Over a 24-year period, from 1879 to 1902, the government established over 150 boarding schools, of which 25 were off-reservation.[26] With the growth in the boarding school system, various Indian Commissioners in Washington began to call for standardization of the curricula. As early as 1889, Commissioner Thomas J. Morgan advocated for the systematization of the course of study: "So far as possible, there should be a uniform course of study, similar methods of instruction, the same textbooks, and a carefully organized and well understood system of industrial training."[27] Under Morgan, by the mid-1890s there was increasing emphasis on military organization; both boys and girls wore uniforms and followed army drills. According to Historian Robert Trennert, "Most school officials were united in their praise of military organization. Regimentation served to develop a work ethic; it broke the students' sense of 'Indian time' and ordered their life."[28]

By 1900 the Commissioner's office was reminding school officials that "higher education in the sense ordinarily used has no place in the curriculum of Indian Schools." School officials had come to believe that Indians were lacking in capacity to master academic subjects and were a "child race." Domestic science continued to dominate for women. In 1901, the newly organized Bureau of Indian Affairs issued a "Course of Study for the Indian Schools" authored by Estelle Reel. The publication revealed lowered academic expectations for Indian girls, stressing instead a "scientific approach" to housekeeping. The course of study in domestic science highlighted topics such as protection from disease, avoidance of unsanitary conditions, and an orderly approach to household duties. "Notably absent however, was any commitment to book learning. In its place were slogans like 'Learn the dignity of serving, rather than being served.'"[29]

Indian Vocational Training

In accordance with the practices developed at Hampton, Carlisle, and Phoenix and endorsed by various Commissioners of Indian Affairs and by Superintendent Estelle Reel, boarding schools shared several common features. In the "half-and-half system" students spent half the day in the classroom and half at a work assignment or work detail. Academic curriculum consisted of courses in U.S. history, geography, language, arithmetic, reading, writing, and spelling. Girls spent either the morning or the afternoon doing chores for the school, such as scrubbing floors, making pillowcases and towels, laundering linen, ironing, cooking, serving, and cleaning up. Older girls might study nursing or office work. The girls made and repaired uniforms, sheets, and curtains and helped prepare meals. Boys and young men acquired skills in carpentry, blacksmithing, animal husbandry, baking, and shop. They chopped wood to keep the boilers running. The students kept the live-stock and gardens that furnished the meat, vegetables, and milk served in the dining room. Because funding for schools was insufficient to hire help, the students' labor was necessary for operating the schools.[30]

The "outing system" placed boys and girls with white families during the summer and also during the term. It served the dual purpose of preventing the students from returning to their reservations during the summer and of exposing them to white American culture. The outing system was the brainchild of Richard Henry Pratt, the founder of Carlisle Indian School; Pratt first placed Indian students he had brought to the Hampton Institute with white farm families in the summer of 1878 and continued the practice at Carlisle starting in 1880. In 1900, Pratt reported that 3,214 girls and 5,118 boys had been placed over a 21-year period. Estelle Reel strongly endorsed the outing system, which she said "places the student under the influence of the daily life of a good home, where his inherited weaknesses and tendencies are overcome by the civilized habits which he forms—habits of order, of personal cleanliness and neatness, and of industry and thrift, which displace the old habits of aimless living, unambition, and shiftlessness." Generally, Indian girls who were placed out performed domestic tasks for their "host" families. At Hampton and Carlisle, there was some expectation that the host families would act as guardians and provide opportunities to interact with family members and members of the community. At Phoenix, however, the outing program became little more than a means of providing servants to white householders. "From the opening of the school in 1891, demands for students always exceeded the pool's capacity. One superintendent estimated that he could easily put two hundred girls to work."[31]

A third common feature was the "industrial cottage." An industrial cottage was established at the Hampton Institute as a teaching tool in 1883 when the school enrolled several married Indian couples to serve as examples for the students. The couples were quartered in small frame houses while they learned to maintain attractive and happy homes. Although the married students did not remain long at Hampton, school officials began to use the cottages as model homes where squads of Indian girls might practice living in white-style homes.[32] Other Indian boarding schools followed this model, creating small cottages to house the older girls so that they could practice homemaking in a "homelike" setting. At Chilocco Indian School, "junior and senior girls spent six or nine weeks in the cottages, where they practiced home life, each girl adopting the role of mother, father, daughter, or son. They rotated roles throughout their assignment to the cottage, so each week a girl assumed different tasks and responsibilities."[33]

Indian Responses

As mentioned earlier, many Indian parents resisted sending their children, especially daughters, away to school. Indian communities and individuals engaged in active and passive resistance. Some tribal communities, especially in the Far West—Navajo, Hopi, Apache, Bannock, Shoshone, and Southern Ute—took defiant stands against compulsory government schooling. The Hopi in the Southwest as well as the Mesquakie in Iowa refused to send their children to any government school, on or off the reservation. Because of Hopi resistance, enrollment remained low in the Keams Canyon Boarding School (opened in 1887 to educate Hopi children). Frustrated officials at the Office of Indian Affairs sent federal troops into the village of Oraibi in December 1890 and again in July 1891 in a show of force. Hopi parents reluctantly but peaceably handed over their children. Ultimately, the issue of whether or not to send children to government schools sowed dissent in Indian communities. In the case of Hopi in Oraibi, the community was split into "hostiles" and "friendlies." The "hostiles" opposed to government education policy were forced out of Oraibi and formed a new village, Hotevilla. The residents of Hotevilla remained adamant in their refusal to enroll their children in Keams; finally, in 1911, cavalry troops were sent in to force villagers to give up their children.[34] Other communities sheltered runaways or refused to cooperate with officials trying to track down school deserters.[35]

Even those who had agreed to send children expressed ambivalence or anger at being tricked or misled by school recruiters. Lena Springer, an Omaha woman whose daughter, Alice, died while at Carlisle wrote to Pratt:

> I had [no] idea of sending my children there [to Carlisle], but Miss Fletcher got round Elsie and persuaded her to go and then Alice

wanted to go with her. It was Miss Fletcher's doings that they went, and now my husband is grieving all the time. I do not see why the government put so much power and confidence in Miss Fletcher, as we think she does no good to the Omahas but much harm. She cannot be trusted.[36]

Lena Springer's letter also points to the fact that boarding schools were dangerous for the health of Indian students. Living in crowded dormitories with doubtful sanitation, students were exposed to periodic epidemics of influenza, measles, and mumps but were especially afflicted by tuberculosis and trachoma, an infectious eye disease that, if untreated, led to blindness. An alarming number of students succumbed to pulmonary tuberculosis, although few died at school, since pupils who began to hemorrhage were sent home.[37]

Once at school, many students, openly or covertly, resisted the assimilationist agenda of Indian education. Students frequently ran away, as documented in school records and letters between students and parents. There were also incidents of students setting fire to school buildings.[38] Other students outwardly conformed to school edicts regarding dress and conduct but snuck away to the woods to hold secret Indian dances, engage in story telling, and to play Indian games.[39]

In recent years there have been recovery projects about specific Indian schools based on oral histories of former students.[40] These autobiographical narratives testify to the homesickness that students suffered and the hard work of scrubbing floors and other manual labor. Irene Stewart, a Navajo, recalled,

> Getting our industrial education was very hard. We were detailed to work in the laundry and do all the washing for the school, the hospital and the sanitarium. . . . By the time I graduated from the sixth grade I was a well-trained worker. But I have never forgotten how the steam in the laundry made me sick; how standing and ironing for hours made my legs ache far into the night. By evening I was too tired to play and just fell asleep wherever I sat down.[41]

Former students recall the corporal punishment meted out for disobedience or running away. Helen Sekaquaptewa, who attended Phoenix starting in 1915, reported, "Corporal punishment was given as a matter of course, whipping with a harness strap was administered in a room to the most unruly." While boys were subject to more severe physical punishment, girls were as likely to be subject to humiliation as boys by having to stand in the corner or dress in boy's clothing.[42]

At the same time, many alumni retain fond memories of school activities, such as team sports, picnics, and outings. Most observers say the boarding school system had the unintended consequence of creating a pan-Indian identity by mixing students from different tribes. Students learned to cooperate by playing together on football, baseball, and basketball teams, playing in school bands, or working on school newspapers.[43]

It should also be noted that a few white women reformers opposed boarding schools for Indians, especially compulsory attendance. Ms. Wordon, a teacher at the Santee School in Nebraska, said that her "highest aim is to fit these boys and girls for work among their own people. We do not believe in having them absorbed in Eastern civilization. We propose to teach the fifth commandment at Santee. And how can boys and girls honor their fathers and mothers if they are not where their parents are?"[44] Constance Goddard DuBois, a Connecticut reformer and novelist who wrote several ethnographies of California Indians, opposed a proposed law to force all Indian children to attend boarding schools. She used an equal rights discourse that diverged from the maternalist rhetoric used by proponents of boarding schools: "No white child can be forcibly carried from his home without the consent of his parents," wrote DuBois, "taken to a school inaccessible and remote, and kept a prisoner under close restraint during the term of his education." She concluded, "Let no law be placed upon our statute books that shall mete out to the Indian treatment which would outrage every sentiment of humanity if applied to ourselves."[45]

Regarding the usefulness of boarding school education, it appears that women who went back to their tribal homes found that the housekeeping and domestic skills they had acquired were not appropriate to reservation life. Without electricity and running water, the standards of sanitation and cleanliness they were taught were scarcely practicable. Those who left the reservation found their training, combined with prevailing racial discrimination, left them with few options other than domestic service. The best outcome was employment within the BIA where they might fill positions as school matrons or clerks. However, neither domestic service nor working in the BIA served to integrate them into so-called mainstream American society.[46]

Sally Hyer, in her history of the Santa Fe Indian School, shows that over time Indian people succeeded in subverting the assimilationist goals of the federal government. Her oral histories reveal that in the period from 1890 to 1930, students resisted cultural annihilation and the school's control; in the 1930s, in response to new thinking in the BIA, the school developed programs to foster cultural pride, a focus that continued until its closing in 1961. The school was reopened in 1981 by the All-Pueblo Council of New Mexico as an Indian-focused, community-controlled institution. The history of the Santa Fe Indian School reveals the ways in which Indian people, through many years of individual and organized resistance, gained a measure of control and self-determination over their own education.[47]

Domesticating Women Inmates

Simultaneous with the movement to civilize Indian girls by instructing them in various forms of care work was a parallel effort to reform women convicts through domestic training. The first step toward the goal was the establishment of separate reformatories for women. Before the rise of the movement to create female reformatories in the 1870s, it had been common for women inmates to be incarcerated in the same institutions as men. In some cases they were housed in a separate wing or floor; in other cases they were placed in group rooms or individual cells within the main prison building. Women inmates served a useful function in that they typically performed the laundry, cleaning, and sewing for the entire institution.[48] In the 1830s, prison systems began to isolate women from men prisoners. In 1837, Ohio built a separate building for women prisoners on the grounds of the main prison for men. The same year saw the opening of a stand alone custodial prison for women in Mount Pleasant, New York. Although female staff were in charge of the women inmates in women's prisons, ultimate authority rested with male superintendents, and the rules, discipline, and punishment were more or less identical to those in male institutions.[49]

One reason for the dearth of separate female prisons was the relatively small numbers of women convicted of crimes in the first half of the nineteenth century. Indeed, as late as 1850, women were strikingly underrepresented among prison inmates. Estelle Freedman calculates that in 1850 women made up "only 3.6 percent of the total inmates in thirty-four state and county prisons." Given their small proportions, officials were loath to allocate funds to build and maintain separate institutions just for women.[50]

However, by the mid-nineteenth century, social and economic changes (such as urbanization, geographic mobility, social dislocation, and the loss of male earners to westward migration and military service during the Civil War) increased the economic stresses on women. Many women were left to live on their own with less in the way of kin and community support. Some women turned to prostitution or other criminal activities to survive. Simultaneously, the development of stricter moral codes for women and the increasing use of social control agents, such as urban police, made women special targets for arrest and conviction on "public order" offenses, sometimes referred to as crimes against chastity or decency. Additionally, women became a larger segment of those arrested for drunkenness and disorderly behavior. Records from Massachusetts and New York reveal that the rate of female convictions and incarcerations grew steadily after 1840. In New York, the ratio of female to male convictions rose from 1 to 6 in 1840 to 1 to 2 in 1860. The Civil War years saw an even more dramatic jump. In Massachusetts, the proportion of women among those convicted for crime rose from 20 percent in 1842 to 37.2 percent in 1864.[51]

The first reformers to become involved in the movement to establish women's reformatories in the 1870s and 1880s often had been active in abolitionist or missionary causes and had a strong sense of religious calling. They joined a burgeoning prison reform movement, which advocated for more humane systems that focused on reforming rather than punishing inmates. Through involvement in prison reform and experiences as "lady visitors" to prisons, reform women came to know of the harsh conditions to which female inmates were subjected. They were particularly appalled by the use of physical restraints and corporal punishment, by frequent instances of sexual abuse by male guards, and the trading of sexual favors for tobacco and small privileges. These reformers created a movement that sought alternative approaches to the treatment of female inmates, one that combined moral uplift and training in domestic skills with the aim of remaking the lives of incarcerated women.[52]

The establishment of reform schools for delinquent girls provided a template for subsequent efforts to reform adult women. State juvenile systems operated under the principle of *parens patria,* with the institution acting as disciplinarian and caretaker. The first institution for wayward girls, the State Industrial School for Girls in Lancaster, Massachusetts, was established in 1856. Girls were sent to Lancaster by court order for petty crimes or moral offenses. More than half of such committals were instigated by parents' complaints about their daughters' willful disobedience, running way from home, or wandering around in the streets. Lancaster was situated in a rural area so as to remove the girls from the temptations of city life. It combined features of the common school and the home, offering academic classes, house parents, and, importantly, domestic training. The law establishing Lancaster also provided for an indenture system whereby girls could be placed in domestic service for a period toward the end of their terms.[53] All of these features were later incorporated into the design of women's reformatories.

Indeed, in Massachusetts, reformers looked to Lancaster as the model of what they hoped to achieve in a reformatory for women. An 1870 meeting of reformers passed a resolution "to urge the establishment of separate prisons for women and an asylum or reformatory for girls too old to be sent to Lancaster."[54] Women reformers argued, and male prison leaders came to agree, that female criminals and delinquents differed in essential ways from male criminals and delinquents. In 1873, the Massachusetts Commissioners of Prisons made the case for women's reformatories by arguing, "Women need different management from men: they are more emotional and more susceptible; they are less likely to be influenced by general appeals or force of discipline, and are more open to personal treatment and the influence of kindness. Individual treatment, personalization, essential to a good degree in any prison, is of the greatest importance in a woman's prison."[55]

In putting forth the view that women inmates required gentler and kinder management, the reformatory movement broke from earlier nineteenth century conceptions of female offenders as particularly depraved, more so than any male criminal. These conceptions had been premised on the idea that women were society's moral guardians and that, starting on a higher plane, they had further to fall. According to Francis Leiber, translator of Beaumont and Tocqueville's 1833 treatise on the American penitentiary system, "a woman, when she commits a crime acts more in contradiction to her whole moral organization, i.e., must be more depraved, must have sunk already deeper than a man." According to Nicole Rafter, the female offender was cast as "the archetypical Dark Lady—dangerous, strong, erotic, evil—a direct contrast to the obedient, domestic, chaste, and somewhat childlike Fair Lady of popular imagery." The reformatory movement put forth a new and more sympathetic concept of the woman offender as, at heart, a sister to the Fair Lady: "childlike, wayward, and redeemable, a fallen woman who was more sinned against than a sinner herself."[56]

Women in the reformatory movement also argued that middle-class women of good character were best qualified to reform other women. In the first address by a woman to the American Prison Association in 1875, Rhoda Coffin declared: "Both common sense and reason teach that woman is best adapted to have charge of, meet the wants, and supply the needs of female prisoners. She alone can understand the susceptibilities, temptations, weaknesses and the difficulties by which such prisoners are surrounded; she alone can enter into the most innermost recesses of their beings and minister unto."[57]

Equally important, the reformatory movement leaders argued that women should be accorded positions of authority to oversee and superintend institutions for women. As Elizabeth Buffum Chace stated at the International Prison Congress of 1872: "If there is any way by which the path to a well-order[ed] life can be opened to the fallen woman, it must be done by a woman. And we cannot do it thoroughly unless we share with the men the responsibility and authority which guides and controls these institutions."[58] Additionally, reformers emphasized the importance of employing women of good character as matrons so that they could serve as models of propriety and domesticity.[59] Thus, from the beginning, the women's reformatory movement advocated for female representation on boards of women's reformatories and for female superintendents and staff.

Reformatories for Women

The campaign to establish women's reformatories was a protracted struggle. Members of the reformatory movement had a difficult time persuading state legislatures to pass legislation authorizing funding for building and administering expensive new facilities. Boards of prisons and male prison officials also opposed separate institutions on the ground that the labor of female inmates was necessary for the upkeep of their facilities. According to reformer Isabel C. Barrows, "The keepers of county prisons (in Massachusetts) made of them servants for male convicts, and said they could not spare the women because they were needed to wash, iron, sew, bake, boil, and mend for the men."[60]

Campaigns for female reformatories most often failed because legislatures were loath to fund expensive new facilities and to grant administrative authority to women. Local movements did succeed in establishing the first women's reformatory in 1873 in Indianapolis, and a second in Sherborn, Massachusetts in 1877. However, over the next three decades only three additional reformatories were opened, all in New York State. It was not until 1913 that a fifth reformatory, the New Jersey Reformatory for Women, opened in Clinton. Thereafter, the pace of building of women's institutions accelerated, with some 18 established in the years between 1916 and 1933, when the California Institution for Women was opened in Tehachapi.[61]

Leaders of the reform movement wanted reformatories to focus on young first-time offenders, not hardened drunks, thieves, and prostitutes. They were especially eager to reach "novices" convicted of "sexual misconduct." The ideal candidate for reform was a young working-class white girl convicted of violating sexual standards—perhaps by exercising sexual autonomy, which was viewed as a prelude to entry into prostitution. Although reformers considered these women redeemable, they thought some categories of women to be beyond redemption. Habitual drunkards and older experienced prostitutes were thought too far gone to reform.[62]

The reformers assumed their targets were white. Black women, regardless of age or prior history, were generally outside the compass of the reformers' concerns. Whites considered black girls to be less morally developed than whites and saw black women as too much like men to benefit from a domestic regimen. Black women convicted of even minor offenses were usually sent to custodial prisons rather than to reformatories. In the South they were sent to plantation prisons, where they were treated as harshly as their male counterparts and forced to perform strenuous physical labor. Under the convict leasing system, black women as well as men were hired out to earn money for the prison system or corrupt officials.[63] Not surprisingly, women's reformatories in Arkansas, North Carolina, and Virginia explicitly excluded black women. Northern and Midwestern reformatories resisted having to take black women; if forced to take them, reformatories segregated black and white inmates, placing them in separate facilities. A notable exception was the reformatory at Bedford Hills in New York. At the insistence of its superintendent, Katharine Davis, Bedford Hills housed blacks and whites together.[64] Nonetheless, the overall pattern was that black women were vastly overrepresented in custodial institutions, whereas white women predominated in reformatories. This pattern was partly a result of black women being convicted of felonies at a higher rate but also of the great amount of filtering by authorities, such that white women committing lesser felonies were diverted away from custodial institutions, whereas black women committing similar crimes were directed to them.[65]

In practice, reformatories had little control over who was sentenced to their facilities and were not able to restrict their inmates to young, first-time offenders convicted of misdemeanors. State laws varied regarding which women were sentenced to reformatories and which to custodial institutions, and courts acted expediently depending on how crowded other facilities were. Additionally, there was no sorting of offenders, so that novices and repeat offenders, those incarcerated for minor misdemeanors and serious felonies, were often mixed together. For example, the inmate population at the Massachusetts Reformatory

> consisted of a diverse group of inmates, many of whom did not meet reformers' definitions of hopeful cases. A large proportion—almost half of the inmates in the early decades of the prison, and between a fourth and a third thereafter—were alcoholics over the age of thirty. Chastity offenders, the original fallen women whom reformers wanted to rescue, made up only a fourth of the inmate populace. The dangerous criminals were either professionals and habitual offenders, or women whose crimes had been precipitated by dire circumstances.[66]

The philosophies and outlooks of women superintendents of reformatories varied. Some favored kindness and providing inmates with some time for outings and treats. Other matrons believed in strict discipline and punishment with prolonged periods of no talking or socializing. Despite these philosophical differences, all of the superintendents stressed domestic skills and moral uplift. The reformatories they led used a combination of moral and domestic training in mutually reinforcing ways.

First, their vocational training focused almost exclusively on domestic skills so that inmates could go on to become effective wives, mothers, or domestic servants. Second, they attempted to shape women to conform to middle class notions of femininity, emphasizing the virtues of chastity, marriage, and fidelity. According to Nicole Rafter, "Whereas men's reformatories sought to inculcate 'manliness,' women's reformatories encouraged femininity—sexual restraint, genteel demeanor, and domesticity. When women were disciplined, they might be scolded and sent, like children, to their 'rooms.'"[67]

Although not all schools implemented all of the features, the "ideal" reformatory had certain distinguishing attributes:

REMOVAL   First was the belief in the efficacy of removing inmates from bad influences. This meant taking them away from their accustomed environments, especially from the city, which was thought to be full of temptation. Reformatories tended to be located in rural settings with ample open space. For example, the New York Refuge for Women at Bedford Hills was located on 200 acres in Westchester County; the Western House of Refuge at Albion, New York on 100 acres; and the Massachusetts Reformatory was located on 30 acres in rural Sherborn. Family ties were also discouraged. At Bedford Hills, letters were only allowed every two months and were censored. Only those on an approved list could receive visits and then only four times a year. At the Massachusetts Reformatory, a new inmate spent the first month on probation, during which she received no letters and was not permitted to write any, except in case of an emergency. She was brought before the superintendent and "directed not to rehearse to her companions the sins of her former life, but to consider that the curtain has dropped upon her past, and that she begins with this experience a new life upon a better basis."[68]

COTTAGE PLAN   When women's reformatories were first established, inmates were housed in large buildings like those found in men's prisons. By the 1890s, reformatory leaders turned away from congregate housing and adopted the cottage plan, a model borrowed from juvenile reform institutions for girls. Women's reformatories built after 1890 were made up of numerous small homelike cottages. According to Nicole Rafter, "The cottage plan appealed to these reformers because it was congruent with what they conceived of as women's nature—too passive to attempt escapes, impressionable and therefore in need of gentle discipline. Moreover, the cottage plan offered excellent opportunities for domestic training, which the reformers came to identify as central to the rehabilitation of criminal women."[69] At Bedford Hills, new inmates were placed for an initial period in a reception building with cells as well as rooms, but then were moved to one of four cottages with a total capacity of 238. Each cottage had a flower garden and kitchen. Inmates spent half of each day on domestic chores and the other half receiving an education.[70]

VOCATIONAL TRAINING   Reformatories aimed at "training prisoners to become upright and competent homemakers. Academic, vocational and religious training were woven together in programs that emphasized conformity to middle-class concepts of femininity. . . . Vocational training at the reformatories centered around institutional chores—cleaning, cooking and sewing—partly out of practical necessity, but mostly because administrators believed that reform of female offenders involved making them proficient in domestic tasks."[71] Even as the numbers of women employed in manufacturing and other industries rose in the early decades of the twentieth century, reformatories were slow to institute industrial training on the grounds that the factory environment was morally corrupting. For example, only with the appointment of its fourth superintendent, Jessie Hodder (1910–1931), did the Massachusetts Reformatory begin to provide industrial training to prepare women to be economically self-sufficient. Alongside industrial training, however, women continued to be taught "thorough habits of homemaking," with courses in cooking, hand-sewing, mending, and millinery.[72]

GRADING SYSTEM   By the 1890s it was common for women's reformatories to set up a system of grading inmates according to the level of "reform." In 1900, Ellen Cheney Johnson, the retired Superintendent of the Massachusetts Reformatory, explained the importance of the grading system for prison discipline. She noted that the aim of prison discipline should be "a change of character rather than a change of behavior." The grading system taught inmates to accept routines "because the things that are required of her are the things that make for justice, for order, for happiness, and for the good of the public, of which she is a member." Describing how the grading system worked, she noted: "The system must be so arranged that the prizes shall not be won too easily. They should be gained only by a constant struggle and constant watchfulness. . . . The rules must prohibit some things which are harmless in themselves, and must require many things which in themselves are not of importance, all for the purpose of securing the unremitting watchfulness and unflagging effort by which character is built up."[73]

Johnson's 1896 report while she was superintendent confirms that the rules and grading system focused on many seemingly unimportant behaviors and minute rewards. She explained that a new inmate at Sherborn spent one month on probation, during which she "wears a suit of plain blue denim, and is allowed no privileges beyond those needful for health." Once she finished probation, the inmate was placed in Division I, and she began being marked each week on conduct, labor, and study, with a maximum of 10 marks for perfect deportment and work with marks subtracted for "misconduct, or lack of industry." As an inmate accumulated sufficient marks to move up the ranks, she was promoted successively to Divisions II, III, and IV. Promotion brought gingham uniforms decorated with two, three, or four stripes; the privilege of writing letters more frequently; joining clubs restricted to those in the same division; and somewhat better accommodations.[74]

Not mentioned in the superintendent's report were the extreme constraints placed on inmates' bodily posture and movements and the grading of "freedom" to move one's body. A distinguished visitor to Sherborn reported being impressed by the discipline in an article the Boston Herald in 1896: "I saw no conversation in the shops, certainly less than in a well-governed school. I watched the women in line, those in the first and second divisions clasping their hands together behind, those in the third folding their arms in front, and those in the fourth swinging one arm free and carrying a book or paper in the other."[75]

INDETERMINATE SENTENCES   The grading system was made more effective with the introduction of indeterminate sentences in the 1900s, whereby the length of incarceration was determined by behavior while incarcerated rather than on the seriousness of the original crime. The gradual lengthening of sentences and eventual shift to indeterminate sentences can be seen in the case of the Massachusetts Reformatory. When it opened in 1877, women were sentenced in accordance with prevailing law, which specified one or two months for misdemeanors. Arguing that this was an insufficient amount of time to effect reform, reformatory authorities convinced the legislature to amend the statutes in 1878 setting the minimum sentence at Sherborn to 4 months. In 1880 the statutes were again amended to set a one-year minimum, and finally, in 1903 the legislature established indeterminate sentences with a maximum of two years for a misdemeanor and five years for a felony.[76]

One ironic consequence of the reformatory movement was to subject women to longer sentences than those of men convicted of comparable offenses. At the height of the Progressive Era, separate sentencing systems for men and women were common. In a precedent-setting 1919 case, State v. Heitman, a female defendant challenged her conviction to a state industrial farm for women for an indeterminate sentence when males convicted of the same crime were sentenced to a shorter, fixed term in the county jail. The Supreme Court of Kansas affirmed the legality of unequal sentencing laws on the grounds of innate gender differences, stating: "It required no anatomist, or physiologist, or psychologist, or psychiatrist, to tell the legislature that women are different from men. . . . Women enter spheres of sensation, perception, emotion, desire, knowledge and experience, of an intensity and of a kind which men cannot know. . . . The result is a feminine type radically different from the masculine type, which demands special consideration in the study and treatment of nonconformity to law."[77]

OUTPLACEMENT   In the 1870s it was common for reformatories to have an indenture system whereby the reformatory could contract with families to send a prisoner to work as a domestic servant for a term not to exceed the original sentence. In 1879, at the behest of reformatory officials, Massachusetts passed a law allowing indenture of inmates. Estelle Freedman points out "The indenture system provided an incentive for inmates to acquire domestic skills. Only those who displayed 'fitness for service' while in prison qualified for placement." To be eligible for indenture, an inmate had to be at the highest grade within the grading system described above. Over the next 25 years the Massachusetts Reformatory placed some 1,500 inmates in domestic positions, a quarter of all women serving time there. Over 90 percent of the women completed their indentures. They had a strong incentive to do so, as an 1880 law made running away from service a criminal offense.[78]

Later, when indenture fell into disrepute, many institutions adopted a parole system in which inmates could secure parole by agreeing to work as domestic servants, preferably in homes in small towns or rural areas. At the Western New York Shelter at Albion, about a quarter of inmates serving time during the first two decades of the twentieth century were paroled into domestic service; of the half who were paroled to their families, many also took domestic positions. Reformatory leaders felt that living in a respectable household would expose inmates to good examples of domesticity and family life and keep them away from temptations. However benevolent the intention, these placements still constituted a kind of involuntary servitude. The Albion reformatory required parolees to sign an agreement to accept wages negotiated by the Superintendent and the employer and to have their wages withheld by the employer except for amounts deemed necessary for the servant. Parolees also had to send monthly reports and submit to monthly visits by a parole officer. Parole could be revoked for displays of independence, such as disobedience, failure to work hard enough, or associating with men. The reformatory thus helped the employer to maintain considerable control over the parolee.[79]

Responses of Inmates

Unfortunately, in contrast to the relatively rich material on Native American student responses to the domesticating routines of the Indian schools, there is a distinct paucity of inmate perspectives on the reformatory experience or their life after incarceration. Glimpses of resistance can be caught in some writings by reformatory administrators. Ellen Cheney Johnson, the superintendent of the Massachusetts Reformatory, describes specific instances of resistance, such as an inmate who refused to eat the crust end of bread that was her share that evening and again the next morning when it was served to her for breakfast. When remonstrated for her refusal, the inmate spoke out loudly and defiantly. Johnson also describes inmates as having a general tendency toward resentment, "over-sensitiveness to injustice," excitability, nerves, and passion. She says of the typical inmate: "She does not readily believe that you are working for her interest. She is prone to think that she is being forced into an obnoxious routine, involving cleanliness, attention, industry, and respect, all of which are foreign and distasteful."

However, Johnson's purpose in mentioning these examples was to relate how these negative responses and tendencies are overcome through kindly but firm discipline.[80]

Isabel Barrows discusses the special success of inmates who were placed as domestic servants. She notes, "Since the women have been fitted to go out into families as domestic servants and have been entrusted away from the prison before the expiration of their sentences, they have proved themselves, in almost all cases, so worthy of confidence that the superintendent is unable to meet the demand for such helpers in families." She quotes from letters of former inmates written to officers at the reformatory. Their letters convey relief at being out of confinement and relate mostly cheerful news about their current life. Employers' letters offer testimonials for former inmates working in their homes. One employer enthuses, "[X] has given perfect satisfaction and is the best girl with children that we have ever had." More cautiously, another wrote "[X] has been a very good girl so far. I hope and pray she will never turn back to her wicked ways." Barrows mentions other success stories of women who married and settled down. Barrows notes, "Occasionally a woman goes out and marries the man to whom she owed her downfall. Others find husbands on the farms where they work." One "encouraging" instance of the former kind involved a couple that had strayed such that he ended up in Concord Reformatory and she in Sherborn. After release they married, adopted two children, and lived in a nearby city, "where she proves a most helpful care taker and excellent wife."[81] Unfortunately, as to those who failed to be reformed, those who refused to take domestic positions, those who failed to become self-supporting through a "respectable" occupation, or those who did not marry and establish a household, we can find no further traces.

The Decline of Reformatories

In the early 1900s, a second generation of women reformers took positions of leadership in women's reformatories. This new generation was more professional than the first. Whereas pre-twentieth-century reformers came from backgrounds in volunteerism and religious work, the "new women" entered the corrections field with an education in fields such as social work, law, or medicine. They were career oriented and ambitious to advance. They were less likely to subscribe to the notion of innate differences between men and women or to accept the notion of separate spheres. Accordingly, they called for vocational training beyond homemaking and domestic service. A 1920 New York prison survey suggested that "Bedford and Albion be made strong industrial training centers and expand beyond the present conception of training women for duties related the household." These pleas had little effect, as, without exception, training for developing employable skills remained inadequate, as institutions fell back on "the traditional standbys of household work, power sewing, laundering, and farming."[82]

Influenced by the Progressive Era faith in scientific expertise, the new generation of administrators incorporated the medical model into the reformatory regime. As superintendents, they introduced the practice of having inmates tested and classified by scientific experts. Caught up in contemporary debates about the causes of criminality, many subscribed to prevailing theories that correlated criminality with mental deficiency and physical disease. Reformatories began screening new inmates for venereal disease and administering intelligence tests to identify the "feeble minded" so they could be isolated from the "normal" inmates or transferred to a custodial institution for mental defectives.[83]

Nicole Rafter notes that there was always a fundamental conflict between the goals of treatment and the tactics of control and that the reformatories never achieved the kinds of success that their proponents had hoped for. The reformatories were also undercut by chronic shortages of funds as a result of legislative and institutional opposition, and the lack of funding contributed to a decline in the quality of treatment. Meager salaries, long hours, and unpleasant working conditions undermined the morale of workers. A final blow was dealt by the economic depression of the 1930s, as legislatures sought to cut costs by phasing out reformatories and congregating women into custodial institutions.[84] Nonetheless, the effort to incorporate training of women in caring work and other forms of domestic labor into the American penal and incarceration system had a long legacy beyond the period of its actual implementation. Indeed, throughout the history of women in American society, one of the clearest examples of how force and coercion were used to track women into caring work was the half-century experiment in combining incarceration, reform, and caring work.

"Americanizing" Immigrant Women

Before the twentieth century, native-born Americans by and large did not view the foreign-born as posing a special cultural threat to American unity. Certainly, some "real Americans" were hostile to new immigrants on religious, economic, or racial grounds. For example, two common complaints were that newcomers threatened the standard of living in the United States because of their willingness to work for lower wages, or that they were inferior racially and thus threatened the purity of the American racial stock. Even those who were most aggrieved did not, however, express concern that the foreign born were resisting acculturation. For the most part, native-born Americans had "a confident faith in the natural, easy melting of many peoples into one." They assumed that the pull of American culture was strong enough that newcomers would acculturate on their own over time as immigrants had historically done.[85]

However, as newcomers from southern and eastern Europe, Asia, and Mexico poured into the United States in the 1890s and 1900s, native-born Americans became increasingly concerned about the possible threat that these newcomers posed to what they saw as a unifying American culture. Even those who believed that the new immigrant groups were capable of acculturation came to believe that there needed to be more systematic efforts to foster Americanization.

Historian John Higham notes that the Americanization movement was comprised of two branches. One branch grew out of the settlement houses that were established in working class neighborhoods in the late nineteenth century. Patterned after Jane Addams's Hull House in Chicago, settlement houses undertook projects to improve the lives of neighborhood residents, many of them recent immigrants. Settlement workers and their allies conducted investigations into the state of tenement housing, health care, local schools, and hours, pay, and safety in employment. Based on these studies, they lobbied for state and municipal laws to regulate housing and employment. They also worked to establish agencies to clean up neighborhood streets, enforce housing codes, protect public health, improve sanitation, and monitor conditions in factories and other workplaces. They also provided direct services such as milk distribution centers, visiting nurses, recreational facilities, vocational classes, and summer camps.[86]

Settlement leaders involved in Americanization were drawn from the ranks of progressive reformers who viewed society as consisting of unequal but interdependent parts that needed to be held together for society to survive. As noted earlier, they supported capitalism but abandoned the older notion that it was self-regulating. They also believed the state had a role in protecting those who were unable to fend for themselves in the market. They therefore sought political means to reign in the excesses of capitalism and to bind the unequal parts of society together. How could settlement houses help bind society together? The answer, according to the College Settlement in Los Angeles, run completely by women, was by "help[ing] the privileged and the unprivileged to a better understanding of their mutual obligations." An almost identical goal was stated by the San Francisco Settlement: "to serve as a medium among the different social elements of the city for bringing about a more intelligent and systematic understanding of their mutual obligations." The means by which this could be accomplished, as stated by California progressive Simon J. Lubin (head of California's Commission on Immigration and Housing), were "protection, assistance and education of the newcomer."[87]

Specifically, Progressives viewed Americanization as a tool to integrate immigrant workers into an interdependent society. John Higham describes Progressive Americanizers as democratic and cosmopolitan in orientation. They recognized the value of immigrant cultures ("immigrant gifts"). They supported expressions of ethnic music, arts, and customs and did not see these expressions as barriers to full inclusion. They wanted to include immigrants in the process of Americanization and took a long-term view of acculturation, fully expecting that it would take at least two or three generations to achieve full Americanization.[88]

The second branch of the Americanization crusade grew out of nativist anxieties about national identity and threats to national unity posed by multitudes of people speaking diverse languages, practicing different religions, and representing "old world" values. Not surprisingly, the first nationalist Americanization programs were launched by hereditary patriotic organizations. In 1898 the Buffalo, New York Chapter of the Daughters of the American Revolution (DAR) arranged for lectures on American history and government to be delivered in various foreign languages to prospective immigrant voters. Other chapters soon launched their own programs to instill Americanism. The goal of Americanization, according to a DAR spokesperson was to: "teach obedience to the law, which is the groundwork of true citizenship." The Colonial Dames organized an even more ambitious and varied program of education in 1904. By 1907 the Sons of the American Revolution (SAR) was allocating more than half of its annual budget to Americanization. Its most notable accomplishment was the publication and distribution of more than a million copies of a pamphlet on Americanism translated into 15 languages. In contrast to their Progressives counterparts, nationalists saw little if any value in immigrant cultures. They championed a national unity based on complete conformity to American values; they demanded immediate Americanization, coercive if necessary.[89]

Joining the nationalist Americanizers in the 1910s were business leaders eager to stem unrest among a labor force that was 60 percent immigrant, joining labor organizations, and engaging in strikes. Some large corporations adopted industrial welfare systems designed to control the work force by tying employment and wage levels to compliance with carefully spelled out routines. Regulations often extended to the workers' home life, such as the requirement that workers reside in "respectable" housing rather than in boarding houses. A pioneer of industrial welfare, Henry Ford, set up compulsory English and Americanization schools in Ford factories in 1914. Clinton C. DeWitt, head of Americanization at Ford, described the graduation exercise that took place each Fourth of July. "Our program consists of a pageant in the form of a melting pot, where all the men descend from a boat scene representing the vessel on which they came over. . . . Into the pot 52 nationalities, with their foreign clothes and baggage go and out of the pot after a vigorous stirring by the teacher comes one nationality, viz, American."[90]

During its peak years from 1914 to 1924, the Americanization crusade was a variegated, decentralized movement involving numerous groups and individuals working at local, state, and national levels. Programs teaching English, American history, civics, housekeeping, and preparation for citizenship were sponsored by religious organizations, church congregations, ethnic societies, civic associations, patriotic groups, and corporate employers. By 1921 more than 30 states had passed laws that established agencies to coordinate Americanization programs, as had hundreds of towns and cities. At the federal level, a Division of Immigrant Education was established in the United States Bureau of Education.[91]

Women were central actors in the Americanization movement. Historians have cited the career of Frances H. Kellor as reflective of the shift from settlement house roots to a largely nationalist crusade during the 1910s. Kellor came to Americanization after a career as an attorney, settlement worker, and industrial safety expert. Higham characterizes her as "half reformer, half nationalist," thus representing "both sides of the Americanization movement. She gave it as much central direction as it was ever to receive." In 1909, with support from wealthy New Yorkers, Kellor established a branch of the North American Civic League in New York, which spawned a Committee for Immigrants that in turn formed the National Americanization Committee. By 1916 Kellor was the vice-chair and effective head of both organizations. During World War I, she headed up Americanization efforts in the United States Bureau of Education, for which she raised funds to establish a Division of Immigrant Education. By then she had become clearly nationalist in orientation. After the war, she was a key organizer of the Inter-Racial Council, a business association that sought to "break up the nationalistic, racial groups by combining their members for America." Among its activities was an effort to exercise editorial control over the foreign-language press through the American Association of Foreign Language Newspapers, headed by Kellor.[92]

Another prominent leader was Mary Gibson, who came into Americanization work when she was appointed to California's Commission on Immigration and Housing in 1913. A former school teacher and the widow of a banker, Gibson arrived with 30 years of experience in charity work and civic activities and, in partisan politics, as a Republican office holder. Because women had won suffrage in California in 1911, she was able to leverage organized women's support to get the California Home Teacher Act (which she wrote) passed by the legislature in 1915. The Act authorized the appointment of home teachers to reach immigrant women in their own homes. She also secured funding from the California DAR to fund the first home teachers. Starting in 1915, she directed Americanization efforts statewide as an officer for the California Federation of Women's Clubs; her influence extended nationally when she became chair of the Americanization committee for the General Federation of Women's Clubs in 1919. She was a frequent lecturer and writer on Americanization. During World War I, she chaired the

Americanization Department of the Women's Committee of the State Council of Defense of California.[93]

Aside from Kellor and Gibson many other women were makers of Americanization policy at national and state levels. Women headed many state and local Americanization agencies, and other women contributed as leaders of settlement houses and women's clubs. Perhaps most directly, women constituted the vast majority of elementary school teachers from whose ranks teachers of Americanization came. At a major Americanization conference in Washington, D.C. in 1919, more than half of the over 400 leaders in the field were women.[94]

The women who came to play an important role in Americanization had been part of the generation of women who developed social feminism, "an orientation towards increasing women's 'sphere,'" which used traditional stereotypes about domesticity and maternal instincts to argue that women were peculiarly well suited for a whole range of public tasks.[95]

As leaders and participants in the Americanization campaign, these social feminist women shared with male progressives the vision of societal interdependency but defined a gender-specific role for themselves. For example, in California women Americanizers announced themselves as "patriots who engaged in 'home defense.'" This definition of gendered patriotism revealed two legacies from the nineteenth-century women's movement. First, progressive women Americanizers defined patriotism in terms of gender: "From the beginning of the nineteenth century women reformers believed that 'home defense' or building a family environment supportive of the social order, was women's distinct responsibility. . . . Women of the progressive era enlarged this notion of domesticity by contending that women's 'home duties' required the transformation of the immigrant family, and this necessitated women's inclusion in the Americanization campaign." A second legacy was progressive womens' conviction that workers' poverty and the squalor of their living conditions were attributable to the workers' own moral lapses. They believed conversely that their own affluence was a result of the morality of their homes. "Because of these assumptions, the women saw their patriotic duty clearly: they must teach all women how to serve as moral guardians of the home. If women throughout the United States followed the example of elite women, America would become a morally united, prosperous nation without class conflict."[96]

What these reform women brought to Americanization was a specifically gendered definition of citizenship. Just as male reformers projected a model of male citizenship as constituted through economic and political activity in the public sphere, female reformers projected a model of female citizenship as constituted through caring activity in the private sphere of the home. Helen Varick Boswell, Chair of Education for the General Federation of Women's Clubs, advised: "Make immigrant women good citizens. Help make the homes they care for into American homes. Give their children American ideals at home, as well as in school. Make American standards of living prevail *throughout* the community, not merely in the 'American sections.' Above all show the rest of the community that this work of Americanizing American mothers and immigrant homes is in the highest sense a work of citizenship, a part of the *national* patriotic ideal." Reform women thus politicized domestic stereotypes of women—transforming images of women as homemakers, wives, mothers, and caregivers into key components of the "American Way of Life."[97]

Immigrant Women as Targets of Americanization

Reformers such as Helen Varick Boswell were aware that although Americanization classes held in schools were open to women, very few attended. Thus efforts should be made to reach them in their own homes. One proponent of Americanization work among women claimed: "the foreign women who are the members of large families and who are shut away from American life by a wall of language—women who because of tradition and timidity will never in this generation be reached by the schools or through industrial organizations—must be reached in their own groups."[98]

A Carnegie Corporation report identified the immigrant women in the home as posing the "most difficult" problem confronting Americanization forces. The report recommended that local school boards hire "home teachers" to instruct immigrant women in their own homes.[99] In this regard, some states had already taken the lead in establishing home teacher programs. In 1915 the California legislature passed the Home Teacher Act, which allowed school districts to employ teachers "to work in the homes of the pupils, instructing children and adults in matters related to school attendance and preparation thereof; also in sanitation, in the

English language, in household duties such as the preparation and use of food and of clothing and in the fundamental principles of the American system of government and the rights and duties of citizenship."[100]

In the view of women Americanizers, the immigrant woman could be helped to create a patriotic American home and family by teaching her better homemaking techniques, enlightened childrearing methods, and sound nutrition. The U.S. Bureau of Naturalization's pamphlet for potential teachers, "Suggestions for Americanization Work among Foreign Born Women," published in 1921, listed multiple lessons on "The Home" and "Child Welfare," followed by lessons on "The Mother and the Neighborhood," "The Mother and the School," and "The Mother and the Community." Under these headings were specific topics such as "opening windows for ventilation," "setting the table," "lunches for school children," "harmful and wholesome comic pictures," "the truant child," and "going to the library." The pamphlet went on to a "General Topics" category consisting of lessons on "Number Work and Money," "Holidays," and "Songs, Stories and History." Last, and presumably least, was "Citizenship," which covered "becoming a citizen," "citizenship of women," "citizenship of children," and "state and national laws about citizenship." There were no lessons on the structure of local, state, and federal government, the judicial system, or voting, which were standard topics in Americanization classes for men.[101]

Even in teaching English, it was assumed that the immigrant woman would want and need to talk mostly about domestic matters. Thus the first 20 English lessons outlined in the Commission of Immigration and Housing of California's *Primer for Foreign-Speaking Women* centered on homemaking duties. After the first set of eight lessons on buying groceries for the family, the lessons moved on to housekeeping. The first lesson in this series began with:

I cook.
I wash.
I iron.
I sweep.
I mop.
I dust.

The English lessons also aimed to teach American standards of sanitation, hygiene, and wholesome living, as illustrated in the twentieth lesson, which consisted of:

We must eat good food.
We must drink good water.
We must have good milk.
We must bathe often.
We must sleep with our windows open.
We must not stay in the house all the time.[102]

Women Americanizers were also concerned about reforming nutrition and diet. In the view of some, hunger and underfeeding were viewed as consequences not so much of poverty (although poverty was certainly recognized as a factor) but of the wrong choice of foods and failure to budget food money to make it last through the week. According to home economics teacher Pearl Idelia Ellis, malnourishment came "not so much from lack of food as from not having the right varieties of foods containing constituents favorable to growth and development." Ellis added, "The pangs of hunger are accelerators of criminal tendencies."[103]

Female Americanizers, especially those in home economics, stressed the superiority of American foods. In Eastern cities, American club women conducted a campaign against cabbage. Helen Varick Boswell, Chairman of Education for the General Federation of Women's Clubs, opined that domestic educators must teach the preparation of "American vegetables, instead of the inevitable cabbage." The Carnegie Corporation study of Americanization cited with approval a study that discovered that "dampness in Polish houses and the tendency of wallpaper to come off the walls were due to the continual flow of steam from the kitchen stove" where workers' wives were wont to cook "cabbage soup."[104] In the West, where Mexicans were the main targets of concern, the Mexican diet of tortillas and beans came under attack. According to a California Americanizer and home economist, "the modern Mexican woman should serve bread instead of tortillas, lettuce instead of beans and broil foods rather than fry them."[105]

Another area of concern was hygiene and cleanliness. A domestic educator in Buffalo wrote that her most difficult task was the teaching of personal cleanliness "because the immigrant standard in this matter is so low." She noted "Some women have a feeling that cleanliness is a condition only for the rich and that if one is poor it follows as a natural course that one is dirty."[106] A supervisor of homemaking classes in rural Arizona reported that among rural Mexican families "sanitation is a sealed book." Regarding personal cleanliness, she noted, that it was not unusual for a "little mite" to show up to school "filthy dirty." Also, even though "A young woman may seem to be smartly dressed . . . a closer inspection will disclose the line where the powder ends and the water did not touch."[107]

Settlement houses in some cities created model flats in tenements so that immigrants would have a "home to copy." In California, they established "cottages"—small houses or school rooms furnished with American style furniture and fully equipped kitchens. In Boston, the Women's Municipal League rented a flat in which social workers from the South End House provided tenants with advice on dealing with landlords. In New York, Lillian Wald and Mabel Hyde Kittredge opened "The Flat" at the Henry Street Settlement. Equipped with "furniture that required the least possible labor to keep it free from dirt and vermin, . . . classes were formed to teach housekeeping in its every detail. . . . Cleaning, disinfecting, purchasing of actual supplies in the actual shops of the neighborhood, household accounts, nursing, all the elements of housekeeping were systematically taught."[108]

Kittredge started other model tenements and founded the Association of Practical Housekeeping Centers. She published a textbook in 1911 in which she laid out a detailed list of furnishings and equipment for a model tenement flat and lesson plans, focusing especially on cleaning everything from floors to brass fixtures and bathtubs, laundry, including preparing starch and ironing. She recommended painted walls in light colors, such as yellow, simple stained wooden floors, shelves throughout the house to hold necessities, window seats for storage, white painted furniture, and clearly labeled jars for staples. With regard to decoration, she noted that "A few good pictures add a great deal to a home. It is better to have these on the living-room wall. If it is desired to have pictures in the bedrooms, a sanitary way is to paste the prints on the painted walls and to wash them over with liquid shellac. Picture and wall may then be washed at the same time."[109]

Kittredge and her followers believed that simple furnishings and convenient storage would encourage neatness and cleanliness, but these recommendations often clashed with immigrant notions of household beauty. European immigrants brought with them tastes from their cultures of origin that associated rich colors, carpets, and upholstered furniture with moving up in the world. If they could afford to, they often purchased a piano for the living room. Americanizers viewed the ornamentation and furniture preferred by immigrants as making it nearly impossible to maintain cleanliness.[110]

Fostering Individualism and Ambition

Elizabeth Ewen notes that reformers became concerned about immigrant women because they stood at the center of an immigrant culture that maintained preindustrial values such as cooperation and the primacy of family well-being over individual ambition. Reformers believed that if immigrant women could become inculcated with American values, they would foster individualism and ambition and thereby raise the family's standard of living. Mabel Hyde Kittredge urged home teachers to inculcate "restlessness and dissatisfaction" with shoddy workmanship and poor living conditions. They should not "accept the fallen plaster, the dish-water that leaks through the flat above and the dirty and dark hall."[111] In a complementary vein, home teachers were advised to help cultivate an appreciation and desire for finer things. Thus home teachers were to recommend that immigrant women set the table on a white tablecloth with flowers and be taught proper setting of the table, mealtime etiquette, and other niceties.[112]

Although the primary aim of training immigrant women in domestic skills was as a means to Americanize immigrant families (especially the men and boys), a secondary aim was to prepare them for household service in American homes. Preparation in American methods of housekeeping would create a pool of "skilled" workers to relieve the chronic shortage of household servants. For immigrant women who did not enter household service, it was hoped that they would find positions in laundries and food service.[113] A primer for teaching English to "Foreign Speaking Women," published by the California Commission of Immigration, had only one sample dialogue for potential job seekers, as follows;

First Pupil—I want to work.
Second Pupil—What can you do?
First Pupil—I can wash and iron.
Second Pupil—What else?
First Pupil—I can wash windows and clean house.
Second Pupil—Can you cook?
First Pupil—I can do plain cooking.
Second Pupil—What wages do you want?

First Pupil—Two dollars a day.
Second pupil—Will you come to my house Monday to wash?
First Pupil—Gladly.
Second Pupil—I shall expect you. Goodbye.[114]

Immigrant Women's Responses

Reform women's efforts to Americanize immigrant women by inculcating the obligation to maintain homes that lived up to the American standard and by teaching specific skills to prepare American food, manage a budget, clean and decorate their homes, and possibly those of white employers, have been documented from their own writings and records. On the other hand, the perspectives of immigrant women who were the targets of these Americanization efforts are by and large not documented. Their responses to Americanization programs are best captured by records that were kept of enrollment and attendance in classes. From these records, Maxine Seller concluded, "Consistently low registrations and high drop out rates . . . indicate that many women, perhaps the majority, reacted negatively." In California, the dropout rate for home teacher classes was 80 percent. Immigrant women did make use of some services such as well-baby clinics, and they sometimes asked social workers to intervene in cases of family violence. Certain kinds of domestic classes were fairly popular; for instance, settlement houses found that sewing and needlework classes were the best attended. The reformers were happy to offer such classes because they believed they helped cultivate both aesthetic sensibilities and practicality. They also found it a good entry point for gaining trust; for example, a class on sewing clothes for an infant attracted young mothers. Even here, however, teachers tried to steer immigrant women away from what they considered gaudy fabrics toward sturdy and practical materials or to switch their interest from clothes to sewing curtains to decorate a house inexpensively.[115]

Demise of Americanization

Although the settlement movement was the first to establish Americanization programs starting in the 1890s, the Americanization crusade became increasingly dominated by militant nationalists in the 1910s.

As noted previously, nationalists entered the field of Americanization because of their fear that immigrant cultures were threatening American unity. These fears mounted with the breakout of World War I in Europe, the Bolshevik revolution in Russia, and the rise of labor unrest in the form of strikes and demonstrations that were violently put down. Conformity, loyalty, patriotism, and 100 percent Americanism came to define what it meant to be American. Simultaneously, many progressives became disillusioned about the war and became suspicious of nationalism, which they saw as triggering militarism. Their disillusion and misgivings led them to withdraw from the Americanization movement, ceding the movement to the nationalists. Rabid nationalism peaked in 1920 and 1921, with campaigns to make English the national language, prohibit private (i.e., ethnic and religious) schools, and suppress foreign language newspapers. Nationalists also fought to restrict non-citizen access to occupational and economic opportunity.[116]

Eventually, nationalists turned away from Americanization and toward exclusion. The exclusionist impulse triumphed with the passage of the Immigration Act of 1924, which severely reduced immigration from eastern and southern Europe and cut off entry of immigrants from Asia. Then, the zeal for Americanization abated, and federal, state, and private funding dried up. By the late 1920s, the Americanization movement seemed like a distant memory.[117]

Reforms and the American Empire

Analysis of United States policies toward the colonial subjects it inherited as a result of imperial expansion in the late nineteenth century indicates that the domestication of women was an essential element of projects of pacification and incorporation of subject peoples. There are clear links between the design of programs to "remake" and reform internal minorities and those used to civilize non-white peoples in newly acquired territories. In a single fateful year, 1898, the United States annexed Hawai'i and took possession of the Philippines, Puerto Rico, and Guam as a result of a peace settlement with Spain.[118] Hawai'i already had a powerful Anglo-American elite, which had converted Native Hawaiians to Christianity and introduced the English language and taught the superiority of Western culture. Puerto Rico and the Philippines, however, would require concerted efforts to Americanize and (in the case of the Philippines, especially) "civilize" the peoples in the newly acquired territories.

The United States quickly imposed English as either the sole or co-official language and established Anglo-American forms of governance overseen by U.S.-appointed commissioners. In Puerto Rico, a combination of English and American systems was used to create a governing structure headed by an American governor, a cabinet consisting of five Puerto Rican and six U.S. members, and an elected legislature. In the Philippines, the United States set up an American-style tripartite form of government comprised of legislative, judicial, and executive branches, the responsibility for which was delegated to a presidentially appointed group of commissioners.[119] The native populations, including the elites, were viewed as unprepared for self-rule and thus needed to undergo a period of tutelage. The stated goal was to grant greater self-governance when the United States judged that the native elite proved they were ready.

An important component of preparation for self-governance was the establishment of U.S.-style public education. In Puerto Rico and the Philippines, departments of education were set up with an American Commissioner of Education as head, and English was declared the medium of instruction. Clearly, the U.S. experience with Native Americans provided a template for what the content of education should be. Some 6,000 extra copies of the Standard Course of Study developed for the Indian school system were printed and sent to Puerto Rico and the Philippines to be used in their school systems.[120] In the case of Puerto Rico, the connection with Indian schooling was even more direct. John Eaton, who had been Director of Indian Affairs and a close friend of Richard Henry Pratt, the founder of the Carlisle Indian School, became Commissioner of Education in Puerto Rico. Eaton hatched the idea of sending Puerto Rican children to Carlisle. Although ill health forced Eaton to leave the island shortly after he arrived, his successor, Martin Grove Brumbaugh recruited students, mostly from elite families, to leave the island to attend the Carlisle Indian School in Pennsylvania, his native state. Some 37 boys and girls from Puerto Rico enrolled at Carlisle in 1901 alone, and at least 60 in total were enrolled.[121]

In the case of the Philippines, American methods of instruction were ensured by bringing in hundreds of American teachers. The first group of 530 (365 men and 165 women) teachers, referred to as

Thomasites (after the ship on which they sailed) arrived in Manila in August of 1901; in subsequent years, many hundreds more Americans were recruited.

Vocational training in housekeeping and household arts was made an important element of girls' education in both Puerto Rico and the Philippines. During the 1920s the Supervisor of Home Economics in "Porto Rico" (as federal officials then spelled it) was Elsie Mae Willsey, who was in charge of home economics work in all of the elementary continuation and high schools as well as the University of Porto Rico. She reported that all of the home economics instructors at the university and the university high school were graduates of U.S. universities, as were heads of some other high schools.[122]

Reporting on the establishment of home economics in the Philippines, Elvessa Ann Stewart, Chief of the Department of Home Economics in the Bureau of Education (1929), noted that domestic training had flourished in Filipino schools for some 20 years, starting with "sewing, cooking and housekeeping." By the late 1920s girls in grades 5 through 7 were required to devote 80 minutes a day to home economics activities, which included "cooking, sewing, housekeeping, sanitation, home nursing, infant care, food selection, embroidery or lacemaking." Efforts were being made to introduce new kinds of vegetables, such as "large delicious, American turnips." Stewart noted that "We do all our teaching in English," but she proudly declared, "all the home economic teachers, all provincial supervisors of home economics, and the general home economics supervisors attached to the central office, as well as the assistant chief, are Filipinos."[123]

As for Hawai'i, there are striking parallels between the educational curriculum at Indian boarding schools and at the Kamehameha Schools, which consisted of separate girls' and boys' boarding schools for Native Hawaiians. As with Indian boarding schools, education at the Kamehameha Schools stressed Christianity, English language, and vocational training so that Hawaiian youth would be trained to become "good and industrious citizens." Vocational training in the Kamehameha Girls' school stressed domestic skills, such as budgeting, cooking, laundry, needlework, and childcare. As in the Indian schools, the Hawaiian female students performed much of the housekeeping labor of the school, including cooking, cleaning, and laundry, so that the expense of running the institution was minimized.[124] The culminating experience for senior girls was living in a practice cottage where, after five years of training, six senior girls at a time spent six weeks living as a family and took turns being in charge of specific household tasks. The family extended to include a real baby, placed in the cottage for the school year. Each girl acted as "baby director" for one week, during which she took around-the-clock responsibility for feeding, bathing, and minding the infant and did not attend any classes.[125]

Reform Efforts within the African American Community

By and large, African American women were excluded from the reform efforts described earlier in this chapter. The Native American boarding schools were focused just on that group, the reformatory movement concentrated on "reformable" young white women, and the American-ization programs focused on Europeans immigrants. Thus, with some exceptions, efforts to reform black women emanated from within the African American community itself. The task of assisting black girls and women who were bereft of family support or in desperate straits fell to African Americans themselves.

A major branch of African American uplift efforts was dedicated to the establishment of training schools and institutes to provide support and vocational training for working-class or newly urbanized black women. One such institution, the National Training School for Girls, was founded by Nannie H. Burroughs in 1909 in Washington, D.C. In addition to secondary schooling and teacher training, it provided voca-tional courses in "housekeeping, domestic science and art, household administration, management for matrons and directors of school din-ing rooms and dormitories, interior decorating, laundering, home nurs-ing, and printing."[126]

A Midwestern counterpart was the Phyllis Wheatley Association founded in Cleveland, Ohio in 1911 by Jane Edna Hunter. This asso-ciation sought to provide a place to shelter young black women from the dangers and temptations of city life by offering them a meeting place, a boarding house, and vocational courses, many in domestic training. Darlene Clark Hine notes, "It is ironic that Nannie H. Bur-roughs and Jane Edna Hunter established institutions precisely to make available to black women training that would enable them to be better maids.[127]

In some ways, these twin goals of promoting respectability and upper-class servanthood may seem to be deeply conservative and similar to the aims of the domestication projects conducted by elite white women. However, there were important differences. Black women philanthropists had a great sense of commonality and shared fate with those they were "uplifting." Burroughs and Hunter were themselves daughters of slaves and had struggled to get an education. They were aware that the derogatory stereotypes of black women as sexually promiscuous kept all black women, including themselves, vulnerable and powerless. By assisting and educating poor black women, Burroughs, Hunter, and other black women philanthropists sought to destroy these negative images and thereby raise the standing of the entire black community. As Hine notes, in a society that denigrated blacks, "each black girl and boy saved from the streets, educated to be productive and self-respecting citizens, restored to good health, and trained for a skilled job represented a resounding blow to the edifice of Jim Crow, patriarchy, and white privilege."[128]

The many parallels in the goals and design of the three female reform projects are striking: the efforts to create homelike environments in which to house and teach women targeted for reform speaks to elite women's belief that the home was the natural environment for women. The emphasis on the character and person of the white teacher or matron demonstrates the conviction that women served as both guardians and models of morality. The frequent practice of outplacement of Indian girls, prisoners and parolees, and "Americanized" immigrant women in white homes as live-in domestic workers reflected both of the above beliefs and also faith in the home and family as institutions of social control over women. The training in skills useful for domestic service had several underpinnings—the belief in the limited mobility and life prospects of racial minority and working-class women and the belief that work outside the home subjected women to moral dangers. Also notable was the emphasis on bodily conformity to middle-class norms of cleanliness, dress, and demeanor, all of which consumed considerable amounts time and effort that, in the view of the reformers, might otherwise have been wasted on questionable activities. Clearly these projects shared not only similar techniques but also common undergirding ideologies.

Beneath these detailed similarities, however, lies a more profound commonality. In all three cases the domestication of subaltern women operated as an essential element in larger projects for incorporating potentially disruptive groups into a stratified social order. In the case of Native Americans, transforming Indian women into housekeepers in the Anglo-American mold was a necessary element in the project of "civilizing" Indians by getting them to adopt the hetero-patriarchal family form and settle in American-style houses on individually owned plots of land. In turn, civilizing was seen as a way to pacify Indians, end conflict, and open up Indian territory to white expansion. For reformatory inmates, training in domesticity was a means to reign in "unruly" women by preparing them to live in hetero-patriarchal families, as wives and mothers in their own families or as servants in other people's households. As for immigrant women, the adoption of "American" standards of cleanliness, childrearing, and consumption was meant to counter threats that alien cultures and languages supposedly posed to national unity by speeding up acculturation and assimilation into the dominant Anglo-American social order.

All three cases also raise the issue of the apparent contradiction (perhaps even hypocrisy) of elite women in advocating for domesticity and encouraging other women—Native Americans, prison inmates, and immigrants—to become more diligent in the domestic realm while leaving their own homes and taking on public roles for themselves. Women reformers bridged the contradiction in their own minds by applying similar "feminine" values and standards of morality, self-sacrifice, and duty to both private and public housekeeping. Elite women reformers brought to the task of moral and material "uplift" a strong sense of maternal duty, often animated by religious fervor and a passion to be useful. For the most part, they held themselves and their sister reformers to high standards of character and conduct, mindful that they had to model the qualities they sought to instill in others.[129]

These reformers brought varying degrees of empathy and insight to their work. On the one hand, their belief in innate differences between the sexes led them to think that they had a special understanding of other women's feelings and needs. On the other hand, they accepted class inequalities as natural and fair, assuming that it was the superior virtue of men and women of their own class that accounted for their prosperity. They therefore tended to take it for granted that elite women would be guardians of other women's morals. They also assumed that the women they were assisting, even if reformed, would continue to occupy relatively humble positions, whether as farm wives, working women, or working-class mothers. Thus, in vocational education for Indian girls, female inmates, and immigrant mothers, they stressed lessons in thrift so that women from these groups could care for their families with limited resources. They viewed training for domestic service as serving a dual purpose, providing a way for working-class women to supplement husbands' or fathers' (inadequate) earnings and filling the demand for domestic help in middle-class households. To the extent that their efforts succeeded, reform women helped to perpetuate the dominant ideology of women's overarching obligation to care and, simultaneously, reinforced race, class, and gender inequality.

4

From Moral Duty to Legal Obligation

It is commonly understood that women do the vast bulk of caring in the family. The pattern is so pervasive that it tends to be taken for granted as part of the natural order of things rather than being recognized as a socially created arrangement.[1] What underlies the pattern is the deeply held belief that women "ought" to care and the widely held expectation that women "will" care. These beliefs and expectations arise because caring is a status obligation of women in their roles as wife, mother, daughter, or sister.

Status obligations are integral to public and private *morals* that are internalized by members of a community and enforced by others in the community. A woman's self-identity and reputation (both in the larger community and within the family) as a good wife, daughter, and mother rest on her fulfilling her status obligations (i.e., to care). Status obligations are also part of *shared understandings* about the social order. Thus women's caring is viewed as an expression of the society's values and as necessary to ensure civilized life.

We have seen that at least through the mid-twentieth century, there was a strong belief among women that it was their duty to provide care for kin and that they should set aside other activities, including paid jobs, if relatives became ill or disabled and required care. Given the many changes in women's economic, political, and social status, to what extent do these beliefs and norms still apply? What reasons do women today give for why and how they come to assume caregiving responsibilities?

Emily Abel interviewed 14 American daughters caring for elderly mothers. Six of the women explained their motivation in terms of filial gratitude for what their mothers had done for them; however, "eight stated that they were rendering care in spite of rather than because of their treatment as children. They claimed that their parents either had given them insufficient love or had entrusted their care to outsiders, such as nannies or governesses. One woman mused, 'My brother says to me, she was so awful to you, why are you so interested in taking good care of her now? And I couldn't really answer that.' " Abel did not probe further, but Karen Hansen, in her study of reciprocity in American kin networks, suggests the power of status duty. Fran Crane, a working-class woman interviewed by Hansen, expended "endless time and effort" taking care of her mother but "insisted that she neither expected nor received anything in return. 'I wouldn't ask mother for nothing [laughs]. . . . She wouldn't do it to begin with. I've been told 'No' so many times.' " Rather, Fran "accepts caring for her mother as her kin obligation, her duty. And as a kin imperative, she fully intends to honor it." In a similar vein, Jane Aronson's interviews with Canadian daughters taking care of parents indicate that they were swayed by an underlying sense that it was the right thing to do. A 45-year-old woman dealing with her mother's deteriorating health told Aronson, "This is supposed to be a civilized society. I think it's our duty to do these things. And, uh, I don't think that most people. . . . I think most people find it natural to do it." Analogous sentiments were expressed by Canadian women interviewed by Judith Globerman who had been caring for their mothers-in-law. One woman explained, "I do it because it's expected of me and that's just my make up." Another said, "I do it out of my own personal feeling of what is the right thing to do. I guess it's a moral thing because she's my husband's mother."[2]

In the case of spousal care, caregivers are often inarticulate and imprecise in their responses, saying such things as "I can't explain it," "it just seemed natural," or "I would feel guilty if I didn't." This vagueness seems to arise from the "taken for grantedness" of assuming caring responsibilities if you are a wife. In her study of English family caregivers, Clare Ungerson asked Mrs. Fisher, a woman who had cared for her severely disabled husband for 29 years "whether she could think what it was that made her help her husband, she said: 'No, I can't. I just think it's my *duty*. I'm a Lancashire lass; all Lancashire people are like that.' " Later Mrs. Fisher said, "I wouldn't let him go to St. Augustine's [the local mental hospital]. I thought his place was his home. I thought as long as I had health and strength I would look after him. [Why?] I don't know . . . if I let him go I couldn't go out and enjoy myself." Ungerson notes, "By referring to her origins as a 'Lancashire lass,' Mrs. Fisher was, I think, trying to claim that her sense of duty was instinctive and that its source was wholly mysterious to her." Similarly, in a study of Italian working-class women, Isabella Paoletti asked 67-year-old Bice about her reasons for taking care of her disabled husband; Bice rejected the suggestion that she was doing so because of social norms, but finally responded, "By my conscience because I must do it because he is my husband. . . . It is right. He is my husband. Why do others have to do it while I am able to give all I have?"[3]

Ungerson notes that

> marriage is regarded as the supreme caring relationship, rivaled perhaps only by the mother/infant bond. Marriage vows (to which almost all of the caring spouses referred) act to reinforce the idea that one of the fundamental responsibilities of marriage is to care "in sickness and in health." Thus in a sense there seems nothing to say about why and how the married carers emerged; they were simply fulfilling their ascribed roles as spouses, and to do otherwise would be to threaten the very nature and continuity of their marriages.[4]

The primacy of marital responsibility, however, is cross-cut by gendered kinship obligations. Thus spousal obligation may be trumped in the case of husbands with disabled wives if there are daughters or daughters-in-law available for caring. Similarly, the filial duty to care is modified by gender such that daughters are more likely to be seen as the logical caregiver than sons, and, if there are no daughters, the wives of sons, that is, daughters-in-law are seen as the ones who should take responsibility. Just as caregiving is "given" to women, it is "taken away" from men by "everyday" mores. Sandra, a 54-year-old Italian woman, had part-time jobs as a cook for a kindergarten and as a paid home care worker and was also caring for her mother-in-law. Asked if her husband or grown children helped with care, she excused their lack of involvement, saying "they have their jobs . . . it's not that they are not able . . . but there is me who can do it. I can handle by myself." In the same way, a Canadian woman teaching full time, in poor health and feeling overextended by caring for her frail mother, explained her brother's lack of involvement very protectively, "But you see he is in a different situation. He's head of a company. He's under a lot of pressure. He's inherited some of the problems my father had physically. . . . So I'm not going to put a load of anything on him."[5]

Both men and women often explain women's caregiving arrangements as "natural," not just because women generally are "more suited" to be caregivers but because the specific woman who is providing care is oriented toward caring. For example, a Canadian daughter-in-law caring for her husband's parents explained "I was always the responsible one, taking care of little kids, always the sensible one, the most competent one. I still am." A son talking about his wife taking care of his parents said "she's the prime person as far as handling all this. But that's her style. She is very family oriented, very emotional about these kinds of things. I am just too distant the other way."[6]

The evidence from these studies of contemporary caregivers' reasoning confirms the power of everyday thought, face-to-face relations, and internalized beliefs about the "proper" roles of men and women in perpetuating and maintaining women's status duty to provide care. However, this is not the whole story. Another important part has to do with the institutionalization of status obligations, particularly by the state through law and social policy. Despite their seeming objectivity and impersonality, law and social policy, both as formulated in documents and statutes and as interpreted by agents of the state such as judges and bureaucrats, incorporate public and private morals and shared understandings of women's status duties, including the obligation to care. They do so by codifying the family as the primary site for meeting dependency needs and by assigning to women, particularly in their roles as wives and mothers, primary responsibility for meeting dependency needs by providing care within the family. Thus, law and social policy play a central role in maintaining status obligations by legitimating them and giving them material force (through granting or withholding resources).

The state has played a significant role in defining and maintaining women's obligation to care in two areas. First, marriage and family law codified wives' duty to provide domestic services, including nursing care. Second, social welfare provisions for dependent disabled individuals traditionally assumed that family members, particularly wives and mothers, had primary responsibility for providing unpaid care.

Marriage and Family Law

Under common law, the legal identity of a married woman was subsumed under that of her husband. In Blackstone's famous explanation of coverture: "By marriage husband and wife are one person in the law: that is, the very being or legal existence of the woman is suspended during the marriage, or at least is incorporated and consolidated into that of the husband: under whose wing, protection, and cover, she performs everything. . . . Upon this principle, of a union of person in husband and wife, depend almost all the legal rights, duties, and disabilities, that either one of them acquire by marriage."[7]

On the one hand, coverture meant that a married woman lacked an independent legal identity and thus could not bring legal suits, make contracts, draft wills, or hold property in her own name. On the other hand, because a wife's identity was "covered" by that of her husband, he could bring suit in both their names, sell or acquire property without her consent, and contract his wife's labor to a third party. He was also liable for his wife's debts whether incurred before or after marriage.

Under the common-law doctrine of marital service, a wife was obligated to provide her services in exchange for her husband's support; consequently, a husband owned his wife's labor and any earnings from it. Although there was no comprehensive or official list of wives' duties, courts generally included such tasks as assisting in family enterprises, keeping house, nursing family members through illness, and caring for children.[8] A husband had a reciprocal obligation to provide support, generally interpreted to mean shelter, food, clothing, and necessary household goods.[9] In short, marital relations were ordered by status obligations, namely duties that accrued to an individual on the basis of occupying a particular position as husband or wife.

Starting in 1839, individual states began passing married women's property acts. These laws varied from state to state, but they generally granted to women the right to buy, own, and sell property that they had owned prior to marriage. By the 1870s, most states had such statutes. These laws were intended primarily to enable women whose husbands deserted them (an occurrence that became more common as men migrated alone to the West) to rent, lease, or sell property so as to avoid falling into penury and becoming dependent on charity. The laws also ensured that fathers could sign over to daughters property that would remain in their family line, rather than pass to sons-in-law; they also allowed that same property to be sheltered from the husband's creditors. Yet the laws, at least as enforced, did not undercut a co-resident husband's control over his wife's property; in practice, co-resident husbands continued to exercise control over wives' property and to treat it as their own. The rights embodied in married women's property acts became relevant only when couples separated or divorced and their assets needed to be divided, when couples attempted to shelter the wife's assets from debt claims against the husband, and, as mentioned above, when deserted wives needed to be able to sell, rent, or lease property on their own.[10]

Between 1855 and 1879, most states in the North, Midwest, and West also passed earning statutes that recognized women's right to contract their labor and ownership of any earnings from their own labor. Some states, particularly in the South and Southwest, were slow to follow suit, but by the start of World War I, almost all states had adopted some form of earning statute. In the meantime, New York and other states modified their statutes to further expand married women's economic rights, including rights to make wills, to bring suit, and to purchase and sell property in their own names.[11]

Earnings statutes were particularly critical to the question of wives' caring labor because they explicitly recognized a married woman's labor as her own separate property rather than her husband's. This recognition would seemingly negate the common-law doctrine of marital service. Indeed, until fairly recently, the common wisdom was that the combination of married women's property laws, earnings statutes, and other legal reforms emancipated married women from the liabilities of coverture by giving married women the same rights as single women (feme sole).

However, since the 1980s scholars have recognized that in the past legislatures and courts severely circumscribed the reach of earnings statutes so as to preserve the husband's common-law rights.[12] Reva Siegel has argued that these statutory reforms actually helped to preserve coverture by modernizing the legal basis for husbands' control over wives' labor. In this account, legislatures and courts together reframed wives' service obligations within the emergent doctrine of separate spheres. The male and female spheres—market and home, respectively—

were construed as operating according to different principles. Whereas the market was governed by self-interest and liberty of contract, the home was governed by altruism and status obligations.[13] Katherine Silbaugh has pointed out that whereas common-law rulings recognized the economic exchange involved in marriage (wifely service for husbandly support), postreform rulings increasingly denied economic exchange as the basis of marital relations by framing services of wives as "love" rather than "labor."[14]

Many different kinds of lawsuits were brought that tested the implications of earnings statutes for whether wives' labor in the family, including housework and nursing, assistance in family farms and businesses, and home-based income earning for third parties (such as keeping boarders) entitled them to a share of assets acquired partly through their labor.

For the purposes of this chapter, I focus on two subsets of cases that dealt specifically with the implication of earnings statutes for wives' caring labor, which courts commonly referred to by such terms as "wifely duties," "domestic responsibilities," "housekeeping," and "nursing." First were lawsuits brought by widows or wives claiming shares of their husbands' assets based on a private agreement stating that husbands or their estates would compensate them for providing housekeeping and/or nursing services. Second were lawsuits brought by husbands claiming damages for loss of wives' services due to injuries caused by third party negligence.

It should be noted at the outset that the litigants in these cases (as well as the judges and attorneys) were almost certainly white. This can be deduced from the absence of any mention of race by the judges, who can be assumed to have mentioned race if one or the other party in the suit was not white. For much of the time when these cases were being adjudicated, blacks and other minorities were denied access to civil courts to seek redress. Moreover, litigants had to have sufficient financial resources to fight over and to bring and defend lawsuits, a condition that the vast majority of people of color lacked. Thus, we cannot know if men and women of color would have brought similar suits if they had resources and access to the courts; nor can we know if the judges would have applied the same standards or used the same reasoning for litigants of color. Therefore, the standards and reasoning can be assumed to be those held by and also applied to whites.

Private Agreements to Compensate Wives for Care

The first cases of wives seeking to enforce private agreements to provide nursing or housekeeping services in exchange for compensation were filed in the 1870s, shortly after the passage of married women's earning statutes. In some cases, wives brought suit because husbands had failed to fulfill the terms of the agreement by not transferring property or making provision in their wills as promised. In other cases, wives filed suits in order to shelter a portion of assets that their husbands' creditors were attempting to seize. In all, I located 20 court cases brought by widows or wives seeking financial settlements based on private agreements for payment for housekeeping or nursing care services in the years between 1875 and 1993. The volume of cases fell after 1940, by which time it was well known that such claims were invariably rejected. Nonetheless, four cases took place between 1957 and 1993.

In all of the cases, counsel for the wives referred to married women's statutes to support the validity of the agreements, causing judges to ruminate over the meaning of these reforms for traditional rights and obligations in marriage. Did these statutes render obsolete the common law doctrine of marital service? Could these laws be interpreted to mean that a wife could charge her husband for housekeeping and nursing services?

One of the earliest instances in which a court system was called on to answer these questions was the case of Grant v. Green, which was heard on appeal by the Supreme Court of Iowa in 1875. The widow of Thomas Grant had filed suit to collect the sum of $1500 for "caring for, protecting, and managing her husband during an insanity of sixteen months." Mrs. Grant had been appointed a special custodian of her husband by the commissioners of insanity of Henry Country and had entered into written contract with the court-appointed guardian of Thomas Grant. The contract specified that she would be paid $75 a month from Thomas' estate for services as a custodian. A lower court had ruled against Mrs. Grant, and she appealed to the Iowa Supreme Court.[15]

Mrs. Grant's counsel cited state statutes that rendered husbands and wives not liable for their spouses' debts and that recognized that "contracts may be made and liabilities incurred, and the same enforced by or against her to the same extent and in the same manner as if she were unmarried." The justices expressed their dismay at the notion that a wife could exercise a right to set the conditions of her services, asking rhetorically, "Would the maintaining of an action against the husband for nursing him in sickness, greatly promote the harmony of the marital relations or tend to increase domestic happiness and comfort?" The court answered its own question: "Surely, unless compelled by positive legislative enactment, we should not place a construction upon the law which would render such an action possible, or be fraught with consequences so disastrous to the best interest of society." As to Mrs. Grant's right to contract her labor, the court noted, "it is claimed the guardian of the insane person agreed to pay plaintiff for caring for him and that she is entitled to recover under the contract. The answer to this position is that such agreement is altogether without consideration. The service was such an one as she owed to her husband in virtue of the relation existing between them. She had no right to refuse to perform it, nor to demand compensation for performing it."[16] The court affirmed the circuit court's denial of Mrs. Grant's petition.

In this case and in subsequent cases, it is clear that judges found it inconceivable that legislatures intended to overthrow common-law rights of husbands and thus sought ways to exclude domestic and home-based labor from the reach of the reform statutes. To justify their rulings, judges marshaled multiple, sometimes conflicting, rationales for voiding private contracts for wives' services. The rationales can be roughly divided into contractual and anti-contractual arguments.

In many of the cases, especially those that took place in the nineteenth century, judges used contractual arguments. In Grant v. Green, the justices took one common tack of arguing that a valid contract involved "consideration"; that is, both sides had to receive something of value in the exchange. The justices reasoned that Mrs. Grant was obligated to care for her husband by virtue of the marriage relationship; therefore, she was not offering any real consideration for the $1,500 she expected to receive.

Another frequently used contractual argument was that simply by residing with her husband, a wife had received support and thus had already received payment for any services she rendered and thus was not entitled to further compensation. No proof was required that the husband did in fact provide support—it was simply presumed if the couple lived together. Another common contractual argument was that marriage itself was a contract that trumped other contracts. Thus, in Frame v. Frame (1931), the Supreme Court of Texas declared that "where the wife is authorized generally to make contracts, she may contract with her husband *only* for such services as are outside of the purely domestic relations implied in the marital contract."[17] Further, the marital contract superseded any previous contracts. By this reasoning, if a man hired a nurse or housekeeper and contracted with her for her services in exchange for property or a share of his estate, that contract would be immediately invalidated should they subsequently marry.

This was precisely the decision rendered in an Iowa lawsuit, Bohanan v. Maxwell (1921), and in a California case, In Re: Estate of Sonnicksen (1937). In the latter case Andrew Sonnicksen entered into contract with Martha Sullivan, a trained nurse, to give up professional nursing and render him exclusive companionship, care, and nursing; in return she was to receive certain real and personal property upon his death. About a year and a half after making the agreement, Andrew and Martha married and lived together as man and wife until Andrew's death on May 6, 1935. When Andrew failed to leave Martha the designated property in his will, she brought suit against his estate. The California Appeals Court upheld a lower court ruling in favor of defendant, stating:

> When the parties subsequently entered into a contract of marriage and became husband and wife, one of the implied terms of the contract of marriage was that appellant would perform without compensation the services covered by said written agreement. The terms of the two contracts were inconsistent and the necessary legal effect of the marriage contract was to terminate the obligations of the parties under said written agreement. . . . We therefore conclude that appellant was not entitled to an order directing the conveyance of said real property.[18]

In addition to citing the terms of the marriage contract to invalidate private agreements, courts usually also pronounced private contracts for spousal services to be "against public policy," as the justices did in Grant v. Green. They thereby underlined the state's interest in preserving common-law constructions of marriage. In doing so, courts often offered alternate or supplemental justifications that were anti-contractual. They drew on newer ideologies that sanctified the home as an altruistic realm where relations remained unsullied by market considerations. Thus jurists denied the applicability of quid pro quo in family dealings.

In a widely cited case, Foxworthy v. Addams (1910), the Kentucky Court of Appeals stated: "It is the duty of husband and wife to attend, nurse, and care for each other when either is unable to care for himself. It would be contrary to public policy to permit either to make an enforceable contract with the other to perform such services as are ordinarily imposed upon them by the marital relations, and which should be the natural prompting of that love and affection which should always exist between husband and wife."[19] A New York Court of Appeals earlier had stated a frequently cited sentiment in Coleman v. Burr (1883): "To allow such contracts would degrade the wife by making her a menial and a servant in the home where she should discharge marital duties in loving and devoted ministrations."[20] This statement was quoted approvingly by the California Appeals Court in a 1941 case.[21]

Additionally, the courts drew on constructions of the home as a "haven in a heartless world," citing the need to maintain family privacy as a reason for courts to refuse to enforce private agreements between spouses. In Miller v. Miller (1883) the Supreme Court of Iowa declined to enforce an interspousal agreement for services, stating: "The enforcement of this contract as to payments involves an inquiry into just the facts which we have been urging as against public policy. . . . It needs no argument to show that such inquiries in public would strike at the very foundations of domestic life and happiness. Public policy dictates that the door of such inquiries shall be closed; that parties shall not contract in such a manner as to make such inquiries essential to their enforcement."[22]

Whereas these cases made clear that wives were obligated to care for their husbands, the question of whether, in addition, wives were also obligated to take on their husbands' caring responsibilities was tested in a New York case, Coleman v. Burr (1883). The plaintiff, Ellen Burr, brought suit to claim real property that was being held by her husband's creditors. Mrs. Burr averred that this property had been promised her by her husband, Isaac Burr, for nursing his aged and infirm mother. The elder Mrs. Burr suffered a paralytic attack and survived for 8 years and 4 months in a "helpless condition," and her care had devolved on her son's wife, Ellen. Plaintiff's counsel argued that the family was in accord that the agreed-upon compensation, which totaled $2,155, for performing such "irksome, laborious and disgustful" duty "was no more than a fair and reasonable compensation."[23]

The court held that because a wife was duty bound to assist her husband, a husband could delegate his caring responsibilities to his wife, and she was morally and legally bound to accept the assignment. The court opined:

> It would have shocked the moral sense of every right-minded person, if he had not supported her [his mother] in his own household where she could have the tender care, suitable to her age and feeble condition, of her son and his wife and her grandchildren. . . . When, therefore, the wife rendered service in caring for her, she was engaged in discharging a duty which her husband owed his mother and in rendering them she simply discharged a marital duty which she owed to him.[24]

With this ruling the court reinscribed the common-law principle that a wife's domestic labor, including caring services, belonged to her husband and thus was his to command. Indeed, in the Bohanan v. Maxwell case nearly four decades later (1921), the Iowa Supreme Court waxed eloquent, going beyond the parameters of the case at hand to declare, "Whatever services a wife renders in her home for her husband cannot be on her sole and separate account. They are rendered on her husband's account, in the discharge of a duty which she owes him or his family, or in discharge of a duty which he owes to the members of his household."[25]

These two statements of wives' duty to assume a husband's caring responsibilities—to care on his behalf and at his behest—is striking in light of several court cases that found that married women's caring for their own fathers or other relatives could legitimately be treated as compensable services. The assumption in these cases was that married women's primary responsibility is toward their husbands and not toward their own parents and kin. The Bohanan decision is particularly explicit in stating that a wife's care is "rendered on her husband's account" rather than her own account. This framing is still relevant in the twenty-first century, as revealed in the simultaneous valorization of full-time mothering for married women living with husbands and the demonization of welfare dependence among single mothers who are not employed. The latter are viewed as parasites, not entitled to engage in full-time care. The major difference between the two situations is that in the first case, the mother's caring is done on behalf of and at the behest of a male head of household, and in the other the mother's caring is done "on her own account."[26]

Given these continuities, what has changed? Late twentieth-century statutes and court rulings continued to affirm marriage and family as a realm of altruism but shifted to a more gender neutral or symmetrical model of marital relations. The simultaneous maintenance of marital service and the adoption of gender neutrality are demonstrated in the Borelli v. Brusseau case (1993), decided by the California Court of Appeals. In Borelli, a widow contended that her late husband wanted to avoid going into a nursing home even though he would require around-the-clock care. The husband offered to leave certain property to his wife if she would care for him at home. She agreed to do so and cared for him until his death. The husband did not fulfill his promise, and upon his death his will was found to bequeath the promised property to his daughter. The Appeals Court sustained a lower court ruling that the "alleged agreement (appellant) seeks to enforce is without consideration and the alleged contract is void as against public policy." The opinion cited California Civil Code sections 242, 5100 and 5132 as establishing a marital duty of support to include "caring for a spouse who is ill. They also establish that support also encompasses sympathy . . . comfort . . . love, companionship and affection. Thus, the duty of support can no more be 'delegated' to a third party than the statutory duties of fidelity and mutual respect. . . . Marital duties are owed by the spouses personally. This is implicit in the definition of marriage as 'a personal relation arising out of a civil contract between a man and a woman.'"[27]

Two main new elements appear in late twentieth-century cases such as Borelli as well as in the statutes to which they refer. First was the redefinition of the term "support," which had formerly been defined as the husband's responsibility for economic provision, to encompass both spousal services and economic provision. Second was the depiction of spousal obligations as identical for husband and wife. This symmetrical framing of marital duties reflects legal and cultural changes favoring an ideology of gender egalitarianism. Legislatures and courts have to be mindful of federal civil rights legislation that bans discrimination on the basis of gender because they would be vulnerable to legal challenges alleging unequal treatment based on gender. By imposing the same spousal duties on both husband and wife, the legal system seemingly has relieved wives from a greater obligation to perform caring labor.

Yet it is noteworthy that almost all of the cases of spouses bringing claims for compensation or shares of estates based on agreements to provide domestic services and care have been wives. Of the cases I was able to locate, 20 involved wives claiming compensation for caring for husbands, and only two involved husbands caring for wives. The case of Ryan v. Dockery was decided by the Wisconsin Supreme Court in 1908. In this case Edward Ryan filed a claim against the estate of his deceased wife Eliza, based on an agreement that in exchange for his services in caring for, supporting, and nursing her she would leave him all her property upon her death. Although he had fulfilled his part of the agreement, she had not. The court's response was in many ways similar to the responses in cases involving wives claiming promised property. It noted that "The plaintiff simply performed duties required of him by law as a husband which he could not avoid or contract away." However, even as it affirmed husbands' duty to "support, care for, and provide comforts for his wife," the court emphasized the support duty of husbands, noting that the reason public welfare required that husbands not be allowed to shirk their duties was so that "society be thus protected so far as possible from the burden of supporting those of its members who are not ordinarily expected to be wage earners, but may still be performing some of the most important duties pertaining to the social order."[28]

In the case In re: Lord (1979), the Supreme Court of New Mexico affirmed a trial court's decision to disallow the husband Robert Lord from presenting evidence of an antenuptial agreement between him and the deceased Bernice Lord that she would leave him her entire estate if he would marry her and "take care of her like a husband would until her death." Lord attempted to argue that he had performed extraordinary services "beyond the normal duties any spouse owes to the other spouse." The court noted that "The evidence indicates that the decedent was very ill during the marriage and that Lord assisted the decedent and attempted to alleviate her suffering. However, there is nothing exceptional or extraordinary about one spouse using his or her particular skills or aptitudes to assist the other spouse in times of trouble."[29]

Considering the long history of rejecting the validity of private agreements about wives' services, it is noteworthy that statutes and courts have for a much longer period recognized private agreements regarding family resources. The Supreme Court of Wisconsin noted the distinction between the two types of agreement in Ryan v. Dockery (1908), stating, "Husband and wife may contract with each other before marriage as to their mutual property rights, but they cannot vary the personal duties and obligations to each other which result from the marriage contact itself."[30] Indeed, antenuptial and postnuptial agreements that limit alimony and property settlements in case of divorce or death were and are enforced as legitimate contracts. The exception has been in cases where the widow or wife might become destitute (and possibly dependent on state relief).

Suits for Loss of a Wife's Services

The second category of cases enunciating a wife's obligation to care involved husbands suing third parties for injuries to the wife that prevented her from performing domestic duties. Under the common-law doctrine of coverture, husbands, and not wives, had the legal standing to bring suits for torts against the wife. In the nineteenth century some states passed statutes that allowed married women to bring lawsuits. These laws seemingly removed any impediment to married women filing their own claims for injuries that they suffered as a result of another party's negligence or recklessness. Further, the clear implication of earnings statutes was that married women who were employed outside the home could establish claims for loss or impairment of their ability to earn.

As in the first category of cases, the question remained whether these statutory reforms repealed husbands' common law rights to their wives' services. As in the first category of cases, courts ruled that husbands retained these rights. Courts established the rule that a married woman, and not her husband, had cause of action for direct injuries to her but that her husband retained a separate cause of action for expenses incurred for her medical care and for consequent damage to his rights to her services. Indeed, prior to the 1950s, courts ruled that *only* the husband was entitled to seek compensation for the loss or impairment of a wife's ability to keep house, care for children, and work in the family farm or business.[31] Additionally, wives were deemed ineligible to sue for loss of husband's services from a tort because they had no right to such services.[32]

In the same year that the Supreme Court of Iowa ruled that interspousal contracts for wifely care were invalid in Grant v. Green, it heard an appeal in the case of Mewhirter v. Hatten (1875). The plaintiff, Mewhirter, had brought a malpractice suit against a physician, Dr. Hatten, who attended his wife's delivery, contending that she had been permanently disabled and rendered unable to perform domestic duties. Dr. Hatten's counsel argued that under an 1860 statute expanding married women's rights, the husband was not entitled to claim his wife's personal labor or assistance. A circuit court had agreed and rendered judgment for the physician. The Supreme Court, however, strongly disagreed, stating that the statute applied only to situations where a wife was "performing labor or services for others than her husband, or where she is carrying on some business on her own behalf; such [as], for instance, dressmaking or a millinery business or school-teaching." The court went on to note:

> In a word, she is entitled to the wages for her personal labor or services performed for others, but her husband is entitled to her labor and assistance in the discharge of those duties and obligations which arise out of the married relation. We feel very clear that the legislature did not intend by this section of the statute to release and discharge the wife from her common law and scriptural obligation and duty to be a "help-meet" to her husband.[33]

The court painted a dire picture of what would ensue if wives were not obligated to provide their services as unpaid helpmeets and then concluded:

> It seems to us, also, that these changes have not transformed the wife into a hired servant, or established the law to be that the husband, when prostrated on a bed of sickness, will not be entitled to the tender care and watchfulness of his wife, unless he has the ability and

expects to pay her wages therefor. These duties are mutual and reciprocal and essential to the harmony of the marital relation. To abro-
gate these duties, or remove the mutual obligations to perform them,
would be to dissolve that relation and establish that of master and
servant.[34]

Numerous cases were brought in every state by husbands for injuries
suffered by wives, usually involving train, streetcar, or automobile accidents or medical errors, of which I examined 29 cases brought between 1873 and 1984. Many of these cases were extremely complicated
as they involved questions of fact and issues of contributory negligence
by the injured party, but all confronted the conflict between wives'
service obligation under common law and their economic rights under
statutory reforms.

One of the interesting issues that arose had to do with how juries
were to calculate the monetary value of a wife's services. Defendants attempted to have cases dismissed on the grounds that what work wives
performed was vague and its value unsubstantiated. However, early on
trial courts established the principle that even though any calculation
of the worth of wifely services was necessarily imprecise, juries could
arrive at a monetary value by considering the circumstances in the case
and their own experience. Trial judges instructed juries that they could
determine the worth of wives' services based on their own experience,
and appeals courts rejected challenges by defendants to such trial court
instructions. One of the earliest statements of this principle was made
by the Supreme Court of Georgia in Metropolitan St. Railroad v. Johnson, in agreeing with a trial court instruction to the jury: "The actual
facts and circumstances of each case should guide the jury in estimat-
ing for themselves, in light of their own observation and experience
and to the satisfaction of their own consciences, the amount which
would fairly and justly compensate the plaintiff for his loss. . . . There
need be no direct or express evidence of the value of the wife's services,
either by the day, week, month, or any other period of time, or of any
aggregate sum."[35]

Over the next half-century, courts continued to affirm a jury's ability
to arrive at an appropriate monetary value for wives' services. In Denver Consolidated Tramway v. Riley (1899), the Court of Appeals of
Colorado opined that "compensation is to be determined by the jury,

not from evidence of value, but from their own observation, experience and knowledge, conscientiously applied to the facts and circumstances of the case."[36] Likewise, in Meek v. Pacific Electric Railway (1917), the Supreme Court of California observed that "uncontradicted evidence" showing that prior to the injuries, "the wife was in sound health, did the housework, performed the household duties and usual duties of a housewife and that her injuries are permanent and of a nature by reason where of she will never be able to perform her usual duties . . . constituted a sufficient showing upon which the jury, guided by their general knowledge of such matters, were authorized to find the value of such services."[37]

In a 1955 malpractice suit, a California Appeals court determined that the jury in the original trial had been correctly instructed "to consider nothing but the evidence and their own experience." It noted, "The value of such loss must be determined by the triers of fact in the exercise of a sound discretion in the light of their own experience, observation and reflection." The court continued,

> In the case at bar, the proof was that prior to the misfortune that befell Winnie Gist by reason of the negligent surgery, she was a fairly healthy, cheerful, normal woman, active domestically and socially. She had cared for and served her husband and children to their health and happiness. After appellant had finished his work on her, she was discouraged and despondent; she could not do her work inside or outside the home. Winnie was nervous and continually upset; stormed at her children and created an atmosphere of unhappiness.[38]

As in the first category of cases, later twentieth-century court rulings moved toward a more gender-neutral model of marital relations involving redefinition of basic concepts. "Loss of consortium" became the general rubric to refer to "non-economic" damages inflicted on the spouses of individuals who suffered injuries as a result of negligence by third parties. Under common law, consortium referred primarily to the right to sexual relations with one's spouse and only secondarily to services. In the twentieth century consortium was redefined to encompass spousal companionship, affection, society, and assistance as well as sexual relations.

Consortium claims are considered derivative of the injured spouse's claim for compensation for medical expenses, pain and suffering, and the like and thus rested on establishing the validity of the main claim, namely establishing the seriousness of the injury and some degree of negligence by the third party. If the main claim is established, a loss of consortium claim can be considered. Two additional requirements for making the claim are that the plaintiff was legally married to the injured party at the time of the injury and that as a result of the injury the spouse suffered a loss of his or her right of consortium. Under common law only husbands were allowed to sue for loss of spousal services and consortium, and before 1950 courts generally held that wives had no right to sue for loss of consortium.

In 1950, a new precedent was set by a District of Columbia court in Hitaffer v. Argonne, which ruled that there was no bar to recognizing Mrs. Hitaffer's claim to loss of consortium because of injuries suffered by Mr. Hitaffer because of the negligence of the Argonne Company. Rejecting the "medieval concepts of the marriage relationship" favored by other jurisdictions, Judge Clark noted, "The husband owes the same degree of love, affection, felicity, etc., to the wife as she to him. He also owes the material service of support, but above and beyond that he renders other services as his mate's helper in her duties, as advisor and counselor, etc. Under such circumstances it would be a judicial fiat for us to say that a wife may not have an action for loss of consortium due to negligence."[39] Other states were slow to accept the reasoning in Hitaffer, with only four jurisdictions (Arkansas, Georgia, Iowa, and Nebraska) having followed Hitaffer's example by 1958. However, by 2002, 38 states had recognized a wife's right of consortium either by legislation or judicial decision.[40]

Social Welfare and Disability Provisions

We now turn to state and federal social welfare programs designed to meet the medical and rehabilitation needs of injured and disabled individuals. Two of the largest such programs are worker compensation, which is administered by individual states, and disability assistance programs, which are jointly funded by federal and state agencies. Both kinds of programs afford ongoing medical and rehabilitation services for disabled individuals, including those residing in their own homes. Many disabled former workers and frail elderly require assistance in carrying out activities of daily living, such as getting out of bed, bath-

ing, toileting, and dressing, as well as functional activities such as grocery shopping, doing laundry, and bill paying. Both kinds of programs
recognize the need for assistance but have historically operated on the
assumption that the family was responsible for caring for its members
and that relatives, particularly spouses, would provide personal assistance gratis. Therefore, the state function was to act as a backup or supplemental source of support for personal care services.

The first social welfare programs for disability were created during
the Progressive Era with the passage by some states of worker compensation statutes. Significantly, the statutes were titled "Workmen's Compensation" laws, reflecting the gendered conception of paid employment.
These laws established public or private insurance systems (funded by
employer contributions) to extend payments to families of workers killed
on the job and to compensate workers for lost wages and medical expenses resulting from workplace injuries.

As in the case of other social welfare measures, the United States was
belated in developing such systems, which had been established in many
European countries in the late nineteenth century. Also, unlike European programs that were national in scope, worker compensation programs were instituted by and have remained the purview of individual
states. The first compensation laws were passed by legislatures in 10
states in 1911, led by Wisconsin. In 1912 and 1913, 12 more states passed
laws, and other states quickly followed suit. By 1920, 43 states had adopted worker compensation laws, and by 1935 all states except Arkansas and Mississippi had such laws.[41]

Prior to the passage of these statutes workers could pursue compensation only by bringing suit in court against the employer for negligence that caused the injury. Christopher Howard notes that in the
nineteenth century, "prevailing legal doctrine was heavily biased in
favor of employers. If the injured worker or a fellow worker was even
slightly to blame, or if the injury could have been expected given the
nature of the job, the injured worker could not recover damages in
court. Seldom could workers overcome these defenses, so they bore the
cost of industrial accidents."[42] Because employers could delay payment
by filing appeals, even when workers prevailed, many years elapsed
before they could actually collect.

In the mid-nineteenth century some state legislatures began removing the first of these legal defenses, that of inherently hazardous jobs,

starting with two of the most dangerous industries, railroad work and coal mining. Together these two industries accounted for over 7,000 deaths in 1907 alone. By 1910 most states had passed legislation abolishing or modifying this defense, and some had instituted a system of contributory negligence so that workers who were deemed to be partially at fault could still collect some damages.[43] As their defenses were weakened and jury awards grew larger, bigger employers had less reason to oppose an insurance system to deal with injury claims.[44]

Fishback and Kantor have argued that although Progressives and other reformers played an important role in pushing for worker compensation, it eventually succeeded because it was supported by major interest groups: employers, workers, and the insurance industry, all of whom anticipated benefits from such legislation.[45] Additionally, popular support for worker compensation spiked in the aftermath of a series of widely publicized industrial disasters that occurred in 1911: the Triangle Shirtwaist Factory fire in New York City that claimed the lives of 150 women, a Pennsylvania coal mine cave-in in which 75 workers died, and an Alabama coal mine explosion that killed 150 convict workers.[46] These events lent a sense of urgency that spurred legislatures in 22 states to pass worker compensation laws in a brief three-year period (1911–1913).

The aspect of worker compensation statutes that bears on the issue of wives' obligation to care relates to payment for medical expenses for work-related injuries. Although the specific language of the statutes varied widely from state to state, most had provisions that required employers or their insurance entities to cover expenses for medical treatment and nursing services. In addition to care by physicians and other health care professionals, most injured workers relied on family members, most often a wife, to provide nursing and attendant care, whether to aid recovery or to provide long-term assistance for permanent disabilities. Family care sometimes substituted for professional or institutional care, and sometimes it augmented it, especially because hospitals and nursing homes often lacked adequate personnel to provide close care and monitoring.

Nursing care from wives and other family members was most likely offered out of love and duty without expectation of remuneration. Nonetheless, it could be argued that tasks such as changing bandages, administering medicines, feeding, cleaning up after a toilet accident, and lifting and turning an adult body to prevent bedsores went beyond the normal wifely services and, moreover, would not have been necessary but for the workplace injury. Further, the very same tasks, if performed by someone other than a family member, would have to be paid for by the employer. Following this line of reasoning, some workers requested payment for nursing services rendered by their wives or other family members.

It cannot be determined how many such requests were made or what proportion of them were approved by worker compensation commissions. However, it appears that before World War II payment for nursing care by wives was usually disallowed. A brief report in the Harvard Law Review in 1926 noted that "Workmen's compensation laws ordinarily provide that the employer or insurer shall bear the necessary nurse and hospital expenses" and that the benefit "has not been confined to services rendered in a hospital, but has been extended to cases where it was of a kind furnished in hospitals and was not intended to be gratuitous." However, "when the service is rendered by persons who would ordinarily provide it gratuitously, and when it is not of a strictly hospital character, compensation has been denied."[47] This assessment is supported by case records in which commission decisions against (and sometimes for) such payment were appealed through the courts.

A widely cited case of the era was Galway v. Doody (1925). Harry T. Galway applied for compensation for his wife's nursing services for three months while he was bedridden as a result of breaking both his legs in a workplace accident. Mrs. Galway had submitted a bill to the employer, Doody Steel Erecting Company, for $220 to cover 11 weeks of nursing at $20 a week. The compensation commissioners paid the claim, but the award was appealed by the employer. The Connecticut Court of Appeals overturned the commission's ruling, and Galway then filed an appeal with the Court of Errors, First Judicial District, Connecticut, asking for a reversal of the appeal decision. The Court of Errors did not rule out the possibility that compensating a wife for nursing services could be justified under certain restrictive circumstances, namely if the wife was professionally qualified and rendered professional services. The court observed that if Mrs. Galway had been a trained nurse or if her care and services were of "such an exceptional nature that they cannot fairly be said to fall within the scope of the marital duty," the employer might be statutorily required to pay for them." Evidence showed that the surgeon in charge of the injured worker had advised that Galway "be removed to his home for the purpose of counteracting a nervous and restless condition which had developed" and that because Galway was bedridden and unable to walk, he required "a very considerable amount of nursing care and attention which were in fact performed by his wife," the court acknowledged that "his helpless condition doubtless required that Mrs. Galway should be in attendance or within call." Nonetheless, it concluded, "there is nothing in the finding to show that the services rendered were other than those which might reasonably be expected from any affectionate wife who was physically able to give them, or that they were not voluntarily and gratuitously rendered."[48]

As in Galway v. Doody, other courts held that care for an injured spouse was a normal part of wifely duties and that only care of the kind a trained nurse or other health professional could provide qualified for compensation. In at least one case a commission and courts laid down even more stringent conditions for compensation, namely that the wife providing care had to be a trained nurse or health professional. In 1931, the Supreme Court of Nebraska affirmed a trial court ruling that William Claus, an injured worker, was not entitled to compensation for the value of nursing services provided by his wife. "If defendant's wife had been a professional nurse, carrying on her separate profession, and was called as a nurse to care for her husband in a hospital where she was employed, or from her work in the hospital to care for him in his home, a different question would be presented. The evidence, however, shows that defendant's wife had no such occupation. Her occupation was that of the ordinary housewife." In her capacity as housewife, the court noted, "The rule is that the husband is entitled to the services of his wife."[49]

As in the Claus case, it appears that the mere fact of being a housewife and not being employed outside the home contributed to courts viewing wives' nursing services as unskilled, and the allocation of long hours of attendance to the injured worker as not above and beyond the call of duty. Thus, in Graf v. Montgomery (1951), the Supreme Court of Minnesota affirmed a lower court decision denying compensation to Mrs. Graf on the grounds that her care did not go beyond ordinary household services and that, as a housewife, she was not employed and so did not lose income by taking care of her husband.[50]

Starting in the mid-twentieth century, worker compensation officers and courts became more apt to view a wife's nursing services as going beyond "ordinary domestic services" even if she was not a trained nurse.[51] To establish that she was performing nursing services and not ordinary domestic tasks, however, it helped to have an attending physician stating the need for home nursing and that the home nursing was in place of institutional care. In 1948, the Court of Appeals of California upheld a commission award of compensation to Ruth Elliston for nursing services to her husband, Ora Lee, who had suffered a severe head injury on the job. In this case evidence was presented that the attending physician requested Mrs. Elliston to care for him at home because care in the hospital was inadequate and that she had been offered a job at $70 a week but turned it down to nurse her husband.[52]

Still, courts were prone to view a great deal of what might be characterized as "practical nursing" as ordinary domestic tasks that wives were obligated to perform without pay and to exclude it from compensable services. An example of this tendency can be found in Klaplac's Case (1968), in which the Supreme Judicial Court of Massachusetts noted that Mrs. Klaplac, a trained physiotherapist and licensed masseuse, had performed numerous services for her blinded husband such as keeping track of and administering medicines, preparing salt-free meals, dressing and undressing him, and giving him massages to aid circulation. It ruled that with the exception of massage, the other services were not medical and thus not covered by workers' compensation; it remanded the case back to the compensation board to determine whether the attending physician had prescribed massaging to aid circulation "knowing the wife was especially competent to give massage, in which case that particular service was compensable."[53]

In the 1980s some courts began to systemize the criteria for establishing compensability of family nursing care. An often-cited precedent was Warren Trucking Company v. Chandler (1981), in which the Supreme Court of Virginia stated that it subscribed to the "modern rule" that nursing care given to a disabled employee by a spouse is allowable provided the care is "medical attention performed under the direction of a physician" and "of the type usually only rendered by trained attendants and beyond the scope of normal household duties." The Court set out four criteria for establishing whether a spouse's nursing care could be compensated: "1) the employer knows of the employee's need for medical attention at home as a result of the industrial accident; 2) the medical attention is performed under the direction and control of a physician; 3) the care rendered must be of the type usually rendered only by trained attendants and beyond the scope of normal household duties; and 4) there is a means to determine with proper certainty the reasonable value of the services performed by the spouse." These criteria or modifications thereof were adopted in many subsequent cases.[54]

State legislatures, compensation boards, and courts also varied greatly in their assessment of how much time to credit wives for "nursing care" as opposed to "ordinary domestic tasks" and what the monetary value of wives' nursing care was. Two cases, both decided in the 1990s, illustrate the range. At one extreme of "liberality" was Kraemer v. Downey (1992), in which the panel for Colorado's Workers Compensation determined that a spouse was entitled to compensation for all the time she was "on call." When the employer appealed, the Colorado Appeals Court affirmed the original award, stating "We agree with the panel that the spouse should be compensated for all of the hours that she provides such care even though, during some of the time, she is 'actively' doing ordinary household chores and only 'passively' providing the required attendant care." It also accepted an administrative law judge's finding that the cost of $11 to $13 per hour (testified to by the treating physician) was reasonable in the absence of testimony to the contrary.[55]

At the other extreme was the case of Jerome v. Farmers Produce Exchange (1990), in which Missouri's Worker's Compensation Commission awarded Polly Jerome compensation for only one hour per week at $7.00 an hour for ongoing care of her paraplegic husband. On appeal, the Missouri Court of Appeals expressed astonishment at this ruling, pointing out that testimony had established the many and complex tasks that Polly took on, including keeping track of Edward Jerome's vital signs, cleaning him after bowel movements, checking for bed sores, and that she spent 20–25 hours a week on Edward's care. The majority opinion written by Judge Robert Berrey stated, "I feel compelled to express my outrage at this decision of the majority finding the claimant requires nursing care of only one hour per week. Not only is that conclusion contrary to the overwhelming weight of the evidence, but it is also an insult to the claimant."[56]

How to calculate hours and rates of compensation has remained a bone of contention. Commissions and courts in Arkansas, Florida, New Mexico, Texas, and Vermont have determined that the appropriate level of compensation should be the state minimum wage. The justification for this low level has usually been that the wife was doing housework anyway and that the care being provided was unskilled.[57] The Florida Workers Compensation Statute establishes a complicated set of regulations designed to restrict the amount paid to family caregivers. It sets the compensation level at the federal minimum wage if the caregiver is not employed or if the caregiver is employed but provides care during non-employed hours. If the caregiver gives up employment, the wage is the "per-hour value" not to exceed the rate available in the community at large. Additionally, the Florida statute limits the number of hours that family members can be paid to 12 hours per day even if the caregiver is on call around the clock.[58]

Based on the sequence of cases described above, it can be argued that workers' compensation became more liberally interpreted in the second half of the twentieth century to allow payment for wives' nursing services. However, it is important to point out that compensation boards and courts continued to differentiate between "ordinary domestic tasks" and "services of a medical nature" in order to define many specific services involved in family nursing care as "ordinary domestic tasks." By designating activities such as dressing, bathing, and giving medication to a paraplegic spouse as "ordinary domestic tasks" that were owed by reason of the family relationship, they reinforced women's obligation to care.

Spousal and Parental Care

A second type of social welfare laws and regulations that raised issues about whether family care was obligatory and gratuitous or was compensable have been federal and state programs to subsidize home care for the blind, the elderly disabled, and disabled children and adults. In the 1950s, the federal government and individual states established systems, involving joint federal and state funding, for providing disabled individuals not only medical and health services but also hands-on assistance in the tasks of daily living, such as eating and drinking, bathing, toileting, dressing, and mobility; and in instrumental tasks, such as shopping, laundry, meal preparation, and managing medication and finances. Such services cannot include solely housekeeping chores, although such tasks may be included as long as assistance with daily living is the primary focus.[59]

State programs vary in the scope of services and in how the services are provided. The main three modes are agency systems, in which a county contracts with public or private agencies to employ and provide caregivers to clients; consumer-directed systems, in which the consumer directly employs a caregiver and is in charge of hiring, firing, and supervising; and independent provider systems, in which caregivers register with a state or county board, which maintains a list from which clients can choose a caregiver, who bills the state directly for her services.[60] Some states offer several alternative modes and allow clients to choose. The most widely used system has been consumer directed, in which the client receives grants to pay a caregiver. This model immediately raised the issue of whether the client was allowed to employ a family member and have him or her be paid by the program.

Some court cases in the 1970s cleared the way for payment to spouses for care out of social service funds. In Department of Human Resources v. Williams (1973), the plaintiff was receiving a grant from Georgia's Department of Human Resources and contracted with his wife to serve as his attendant to provide domestic and personal care. The Department of Human Services reduced his grant on the theory that he was entitled to his wife's services. Williams appealed this reduction. The court determined that the ruling regarding wives' obligatory services applied only to ordinary household duties, not the extensive personal care of a brain-damaged patient. The court noted also that Mrs. Williams had given up employment to which she was legally entitled to provide the care based on the state's earnings law. The court concluded that the plaintiff's expenditure of grant funds to pay his wife for care was legitimate.[61] Another important case was Vincent v. State of California (1971), in which the California Court of Appeals overturned a decision by the state's Aid to Totally Disabled program to discontinue payment for care by Vincent's wife. The court noted that two other state programs, Old Age Assistance and Aid to the Blind, allowed such payment. It reasoned that the legal obligation of one spouse to care for the other was equally applicable to the three programs and that the difference in policy violated the Equal Protection Clause of the Fourteenth Amendment by treating individuals with similar needs unequally with respect to benefits. In its ruling the court seemed to recognize that spouses can be paid to provide care even though they are also obligated to provide it.[62]

A number of federal programs now subsidize personal care services, including the Veterans Health Administration, but the largest by far is Medicaid, which, starting in 1975, authorized states to exercise a Personal Care Services Option for those eligible under state Medicaid, with half of the costs paid by federal funds and the rest by state and county funds.[63] As of 2004, 30 states and the District of Columbia offered the Personal Services Options as a benefit.[64] The economic rationale for public funding of these services is that many disabled individuals can avoid being institutionalized, which would be far more costly.

Individual states are given wide latitude in defining the kind, amount, and scope of services and in how these services are provided, but there are also some restrictions. One constraint that is relevant to the issue of family care is that "legally responsible relatives," normally interpreted as spouses and parents of minor children, cannot be reimbursed by Medicaid funds.[65] Thus states that wish to allow reimbursement to spouses and parents must foot the entire cost of such reimbursements.

California, the largest state system, has covered payment to family caregivers as part of the In Home Support Services (IHSS) program since the 1970s. A state budget crisis in 1992 impelled Governor Pete Wilson to seek matching Medicaid funds for IHSS. Medicaid, however, would not allow caregiver payments to parents and spouses. Because there was a great deal of popular and political support—thanks to an active and visible disability community—for continuing reimbursements to parents caring for severely disabled children, the IHSS was split into two programs. The Personal Care Services Program, eligible for 50 percent matching funds from Medicaid, did not allow reimbursement for spouses and parents of minor children. The "Residual Program," funded solely by state and county funds, allowed such reimbursement. In order to qualify, parents had to show they were precluded from working full-time because of the severity of the disability, the complicated needs of the child, and the lack of alternative care options. Spouses were covered based on the client's right to decide who would provide the most intimate care needs, toileting and bathing. To be re-imbursed for other services such as transportation to medical appoint-ments or protective supervision, caregivers had to demonstrate they were precluded from working by the demands of caregiving. As of 2003, 81 percent of those receiving personal care services in California did so under the Personal Care Services Program, 15 percent did so under the Residual Program, and 4 percent did so through a combination of the two programs.[66]

When Governor Arnold Schwarzenegger proposed a budget for 2004–2005 that eliminated the Residual Program, it led to a huge out-cry by advocates for the elderly and disabled, health care organizations, and other influential groups. In response, Schwarzenegger, a Republi-can, announced in April 2004 that he was rescinding cuts to the Re-sidual Program and was applying for a federal waiver to allow Medicaid funding of the Residual program. In July 2004, the Republican-controlled federal government approved a "demonstration waiver" with an August 2004 start date and July 2009 expiry date. The waiver programs were so-named because they temporarily removed some of the statutory lim-its of Medicaid, the key one in this instance being the prohibition against hiring spouses and parents of minor clients to provide services. A 2008 study showed that the proportion of "responsible relatives," that is, parents of minor children and spouses of disabled or elderly adults, providing reimbursed care remained constant before and after institution of the Waiver-Plus program.[67] (In 2009, in an effort to pre-pare the public for a cutoff of funding for home care services, Governor Schwarzenegger claimed that these programs were filled with fraudu-lent claims; when challenged by elderly and disabled advocates to back up his statement, it turned out that there was no proof for accusations of widespread fraud. Nonetheless, the governor's budget eliminated almost all state funding for home-care services.)

Unlike worker compensation programs where there are powerful in-terest groups (employers and insurers) constantly challenging awards, assistance programs for disabled and elderly do not have specific inter-est groups fighting against payments for such services. Indeed, there are influential interest groups that support caring for the disabled and elderly in their own homes. The disabled and their advocates, including medical and health professionals and organizations, point out that care that helps people stay in their own homes is less costly than institutionalization. As for paying family members, proponents argue that family members know the client already and are more likely to understand his or her preferences with regard to assistance. Moreover, there is a serious shortage of paid caregivers as well as high rates of turnover, especially given the arduous nature of the work, low wages, and lack of benefits. Proponents of compensating family caregivers argue that family caregivers can help ease the shortage and maintain continuity of care.[68]

One might therefore expect little opposition to reimbursing family members for caring for elderly and disabled people. Yet, there lingers a sense of moral unease with paying family members to care for one another in some quarters. The ideology of separate spheres still has the power to make the introduction of market values into a family relationship appear to be unseemly. Critics of paid care argue that it is irresponsible to spend public funds on services that family members are supposed to provide for free and that compensation will undermine the sense of family obligation. Other concerns are that compensation will attract greedy relatives who will not actually provide adequate care and that close family relationships will make it harder for clients to retain autonomy, report abuse or neglect, or fire a caregiver.[69]

There has been sufficient interest in testing these contentions that state and federal agencies have funded demonstration projects in Ohio, Michigan, California, Arkansas, New Jersey, New York, Florida, and Illinois, comparing agency-directed and client-directed care and, within client-directed care, family and non-family paid caregiving. These studies have found that paid family care generates higher levels of satisfaction among both clients and caregivers and no higher incidence of fraud, abuse, neglect, or unreliability than non-family home care. This is true even though levels of payment are generally well below what one could earn in a full-time job.[70]

Despite research showing that family care is in fact less problematic from the point of view of the welfare of the care receiver, and certainly less costly to the public purse, the Medicaid restrictions against reimbursing "responsible relatives" have remained in place. Most states that exercise the Personal Care Option permit reimbursements to relatives other than spouses and parents of dependent children. According to a 2003 survey by AARP (the organization formerly known as the American Association of Retired Persons), out of 24 state Personal Care programs that responded, 18 allowed such reimbursements.[71] However, some states set even stricter rules that prohibited a larger circle of kin from being reimbursed. Montana's program disallowed payments not only to spouses but also to children (whether natural or adopted), siblings, in-laws, grandparents, and grandchildren.[72] Maryland's program notes on its website that a provider "must not be the spouse, child, parent, sibling, in-law, or have a 'step relationship' to the recipient."[73]

We have come a long way since the 1875 case of Grant v. Green, in which Iowa courts ruled that Rebecca Green was not entitled to compensation for caring for her insane husband as specified in a contract between her and the state commission on the insane. The grounds for the denial were that a husband was entitled to a wife's services by reason of the marriage relationship and thus could not be contracted. A court case a century later illustrates how law and social policy have changed in some ways and not in others. Recall the 1971 case Department of Human Resources v. Williams, in which a Georgia court agreed with the Department of Human Resources' contention that a wife did indeed owe her husband domestic services. However, the court recognized that such obligatory services did not include the extensive personal services required by a brain-damaged patient. Furthermore, it noted, Mrs. Williams had given up employment to care for her husband. Therefore, it concluded, Mr. Williams was entitled to use his grant from the Department of Human Resources to pay his wife to act as his attendant.

By comparing the Grant and Williams decisions, we can see progress toward recognizing some limits to wives' caring obligations, namely that it does not include the kind of extensive care required by a brain-damaged patient. By that standard, Rebecca Green's care for her husband would be deemed well beyond what she was obligated to do as a wife.

At the same time, however, the Williams court's need to further justify the compensation by referring to the wife's loss of paid employment reinscribed the divide between unpaid caring and paid employment. Relying on lost employment and earnings to argue for the validity of compensation has profound gender implications. In the discussion on the California program it was noted that to qualify for reimbursement spouses and parents of minors had to show to varying degrees that they were precluded from full-time employment by their care responsibilities. Using whether or not the caregiver would otherwise be employed in the labor market as a criterion creates the possibility of gender bias in awarding compensation. Stay-at-home wives and mothers would be disqualified by definition, and spouses with interrupted job histories or part-time employment—most likely to be women—would be disadvantaged. A report comparing home-care programs noted that the Texas program confirms this line of reasoning; the author wrote, "Parents (of adult consumers) providing PAS [Personal Assistance Services] prior to program enrollment may be paid with Medicaid funds if the caseworker determines that the parent would otherwise be employed." One advocate pointed to "sexism in (the) decision making process for some caseworkers: fathers may become paid providers but mothers are expected to provide PAS without reimbursement."[74]

A further point is that the Williams decision, as well as many other late twentieth-century cases, continued to differentiate between "skilled nursing care" and "ordinary domestic duties." For example, in 1994, the Supreme Court of Virginia affirmed a lower court decision denying June Dade's claim for $69,000 from her husband Thomas's estate for nursing services prior to his death from encephalitis contracted during hospitalization. The court ruled against June, citing worker compensation rules that provided compensation only if the "care is of a sort normally provided by trained attendants and beyond the scope of normal household duties."[75] The dichotomy between skilled nursing and ordinary domestic duties serves to deskill caring. In turn, the characterization of caring work as unskilled serves to justify the meager compensation offered to family caregivers. Thus, according to a 50-state survey in 2008, the median hourly wage for personal and home care services nationally was $8.54. When adjusted for inflation, median wages fell 4 percent between 1999 and 2006. In 29 states, the median hourly wage was inadequate for an adult with children to survive and was low enough to qualify households for state and local assistance programs.[76]

These restrictions and caveats speak of a continuing desire to preserve the family as a private protected space. There is thus a sense of unease with introducing market relations into the family because the two are seen as diametrically opposed. The demonstration projects on paid family care indicate that conceiving of women's caring as a moral obligation and as deserving of financial compensation are not mutually exclusive. After all, caring for disabled and elderly people benefits not only a specific individual or family but the community and the economy as a whole. Recognition and support of such caring through direct payment acknowledges the contribution to public welfare and the larger economy.

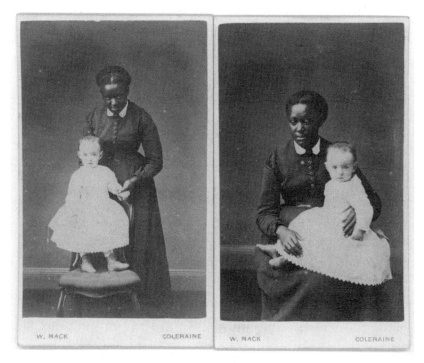

1. Many thousands of female slaves were forced to care for the children of their slave masters and mistresses during the more than 200 years of slavery in the United States. "The Black Nanny." Permission for use from Rob Oechsle (contact@t-enami.org). Uploaded to flickr on August 1, 2008.

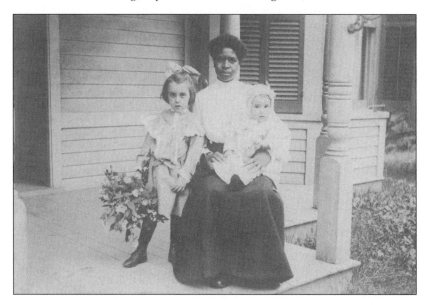

2. Continuing the legacy of slavery, a leading job category for African American women in the late nineteenth and twentieth centuries was "nanny" for white children. Photographs and Prints Division, Schomburg Center for Research in Black Culture, The New York Public Library, Astor, Lenox and Tilden Foundations.

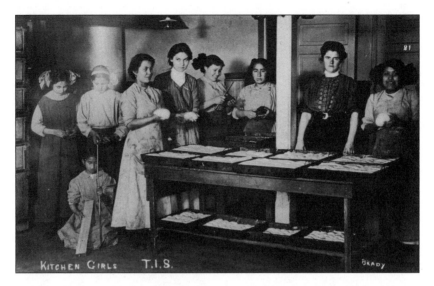

3. Official U.S. policy toward Native American women in the early twentieth century was to force them to abandon traditional Indian ways in favor of becoming "American." "Kitchen girls, Tulalip Indian School, ca. 1912." Museum of History & Industry, Seattle.

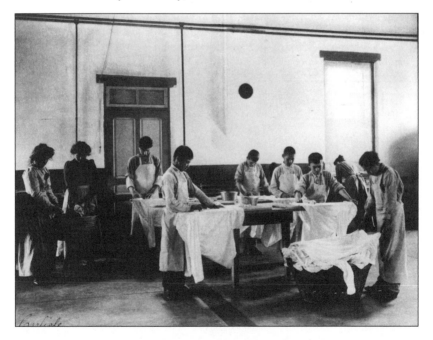

4. Native American girls were often taken away from their families so they could be trained as domestic workers at special institutions, such as the Carlisle Indian School. "Laundry class, Carlisle Indian School, Carlisle, Pennsylvania." Photographer: Frances Benjamin Johnston, Library of Congress Prints and Photographs Division. Non-restricted.

STATE INDUSTRIAL SCHOOL FOR GIRLS
AT LANCASTER

THE IRONING ROOM AT LANCASTER.

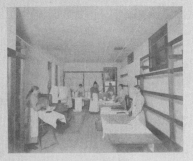

RELEASE ON PROBATION.

After about 18 months a girl of average intelligence is ready to be placed on probation in her own home or in some other family

She still remains under the care of the school until she is 21, and she may be recalled to the school, either for misconduct, or on account of illness or change of place.

LENGTH OF TRAINING IN SCHOOL before placed out on **PROBATION FIRST TIME**

Going home   16 girls, average 1 yr. 6 mos. 5 days
Going to a place, 45 ,,   ,,   1 ,, 9 ,, 5 ,,

LENGTH OF TRAINING IN SCHOOL before 45 girls who had been recalled for unsatisfactory or for unchaste conduct were again **PLACED ON PROBATION**   Average 3 months, 3 days.

Number of **RELOCATIONS** of girls

114	were re-located	once
44	,, ,,	twice
12	,, ,,	three times
4	,, ,,	four ,,
2	,, ,,	five ,,
176	,, ,,	264 ,,

5. "Fallen women" (prisoners) were trained to be care workers, mostly for well-to-do white families. At the Lancaster Industrial School, girls and women were trained to work in "plain, country homes" rather than in homes with luxuries such as electricity and steam heat. "Lancaster State Industrial School for Girls: State Industrial School for Girls at Lancaster: The Girls at Work. Home Making, c. 1900." Unidentified artist. Untitled (Crime, Children: The Ironing Room at State Industrial School for Girls at Lancaster, Massachusetts), c. 1903. Harvard Art Museum, Fogg Art Museum, on deposit from the Carpenter Center for the Visual Arts, Social Museum Collection, 3.202.503. Photo: Imaging Department, copyright President and Fellows of Harvard College.

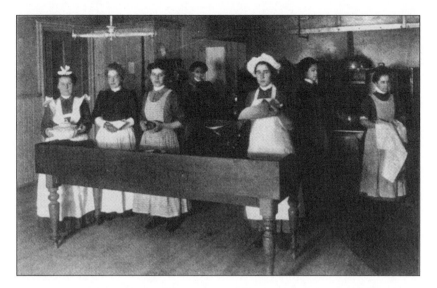

6. Women and girls found guilty of crimes, and of sins such as "disobedience," were incarcerated in reformatories and taught cooking skills so they could get jobs appropriate to their low status upon release. "The Andrew Mercer Reformatory in Toronto, c. 1900." Archives of Ontario, Annual Report of the Inspector of Prisons and Public Charities, Sessional Papers 35 (1903), 87.

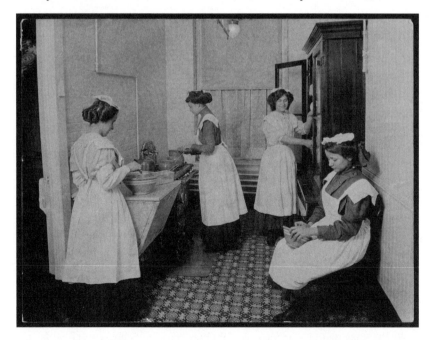

7. The "Americanization" movement focused on turning immigrant women into "typical" stay-at-home wives and mothers, able to care for children, the elderly, and the disabled. "Italian House, Children's Aid Society—Instruction in Homemaking. (The young men who win the graduates of this cooking-class are insured against indigestion.)" Underwood and Underwood, Held at Widener Library. Photo: Imaging Department, copyright President and Fellows of Harvard College.

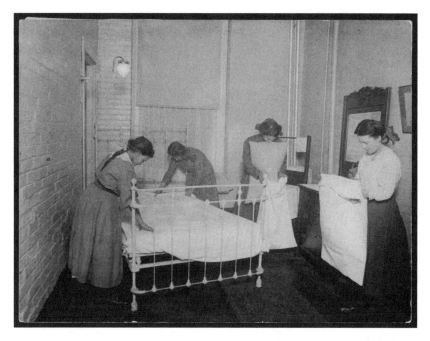

8. Women from "backward" countries such as Italy (shown here) and Ireland were seen as impeding their husbands' and sons' progress, so were trained in "proper" domestic skills. "Italian House, Children's Aid Society—Instruction in Homemaking. Chamber Work in the $120 Model Flat." Underwood and Underwood, Held at Widener Library. Photo: Imaging Department, copyright President and Fellows of Harvard College.

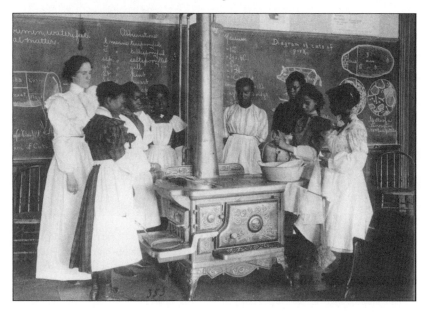

9. Public schools for African Americans had model kitchens so that girls could be trained for jobs as cooks and domestic workers for white families. "African American Schoolgirls with Teacher, Learning to Cook on a Wood Stove in Classroom, 1899?" Photographer: Frances Benjamin Johnston, Library of Congress Prints and Photographs Division. Non-restricted.

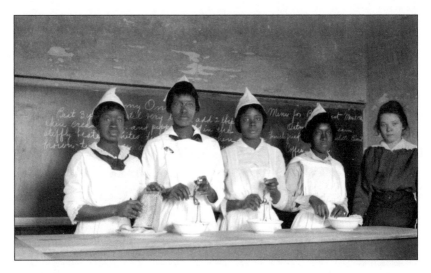

10. African American girls were trained on "modern appliances" such as egg beaters and graters. "Pickens County Training School." The Jackson Davis Collection, Special Collections Department, University of Virginia Library.

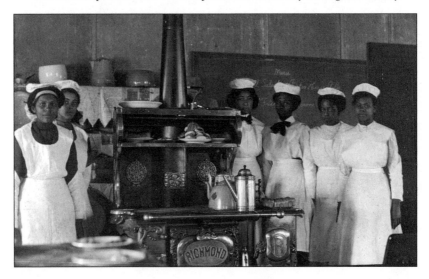

11. African American women were forced into long hours of caring work for white families and in institutional settings, regardless of their own children's needs for care. "Cooking Classes." The Jackson Davis Collection, Special Collections Department, University of Virginia Library.

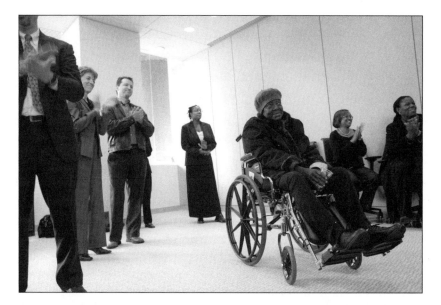

12. Denied equal rights by U.S. labor laws that discriminate against care workers, Evelyn Coke, who worked for a profit-making care-work corporation, sued for minimum wage and overtime pay guaranteed to virtually all other American workers. On the day her case went before the U.S. Supreme Court, Coke was honored at a reception at the Service Employees International Union in Washington, D.C. The Supreme Court ruled against Coke in June 2007. "On the day her case went before the Supreme Court seeking minimum wage and overtime coverage, Evelyn Coke, 73, was honored at a reception at the Service Employees International Union building in Washington." Andrew Councill, for the *New York Times*. Copyright, The New York Times.

5

Paid Caring in the Home

On June 12, 2007, the U.S. Supreme Court unanimously ruled that 73-year-old Evelyn Coke, a Jamaican immigrant who had been employed by a for-profit company, Long Island Care at Home, Ltd., to care for elderly clients in their own homes, was not entitled to back payment of minimum wage and overtime pay. Now retired, Ms. Coke had often worked up to 70 hours a week during her 20-year career. Now disabled herself and in a wheelchair, Ms. Coke required dialysis three times a week. Listening to arguments during the testimony phase in April, she said, "I hope they try to help me because I need help bad."[1] None of the justices were focused on her plight, however. Justice Stephen Breyer instead expressed concerns of families of those she cared for. He worried aloud, "If you win this case, it seems to me suddenly there will be millions of people who will be unable to do it and hence, millions of sick people will move to institutions."[2]

How is it that the federal government and the courts, which express concern about the elderly and the need to keep them out of institutions, also say that the very people who take care of the needs of the elderly and help to keep them out of institutions are not entitled to the same legal protections as most other workers? How is that an employer, in this case a profit-making company, does not have to adhere to the nation's hour and wage standards? To answer these questions, we need to trace the history of legal and governmental policy approaches to paid home care in relation to the overall trend toward "modernization" of labor relations. This history is intertwined with those of marriage and family relations, which have been ruled by status obligations, and that of racialized servitude (indenture and slavery), which has come under principles of property ownership.

With regard to marriage and family relations, up through the mid-twentieth century courts maintained the doctrine of "marital service" in the face of statutory reforms that gave married women rights to contract their own labor. They did so by defining the family and household as a place of refuge from market relations and therefore as governed by status obligations rather than by contract. This belief in the special character of "the home" had profound implications for the treatment of paid care work. Legislatures and courts have dealt with paid care workers as though they are quasi-family members rather than as fully autonomous workers. And, because they have walled off the private household as off limits to public regulation, they have taken a hands-off approach to domestic employment, including home care.

With regard to racialized servitude, through the mid-twentieth century, courts, as well as customs and mores, continued to protect the property interest of employers in the labor of racialized workers despite the banning of formal indenture and chattel slavery. Blacks, Latinos, and Asian immigrants working in primary industries (agriculture and extraction) were subject to coercion and intimidation through such mechanisms as debt bondage, sharecropping, convict labor systems, and violence. Racist ideology justified coercion by negating the personhood of people of color, thus rendering them and their labor "at the disposal" of whites and employers.[3] These assumptions have lingered in the treatment of household domestic and care employees as "hired property."

Overall, then, the state (representing the interests of employers and property owners) has treated relations between employers and domestic employees as a combination of traditional status relations and property relations. The employer is assumed to be entitled to the services of the employee at whatever time the employer wants him or her, and the employee is assumed to be obligated to be available at any time to do whatever is asked. This stands in contrast to the ideal of contractual relations in which rights and duties are delimited by contractual provisions and public regulation. Consequently, labor law has excluded home-care workers from the benefits and protections accorded to other types of workers. The lack of such protections, coupled with the isolated nature of private household labor, has left home-care workers vulnerable to conditions of de facto servitude.

In so arguing, I draw attention to struggles over the cultural meanings of home, care, and labor. Although the exclusion of home-care work from labor law can be analyzed in terms of the power and influence of vested economic interests, it also needs to be analyzed in terms of ideology—beliefs, values, and ideas that make the exclusion appear to be just, fair, even commonsensical. Thus struggles for inclusion have to challenge the ideologies that buttress exclusion. Analysis of legislative debates, administrative language, and court rulings reveals the prevailing assumptions, attitudes, and beliefs about the separation of home and market, the nature and value of care labor, and gender, race, and class relations.

From Master–Servant Laws to Free-Labor Doctrine

The histories of unpaid family care and paid caring started from the same roots. In the colonial period and the early years of the U.S. republic, marital or family relations and labor relations were governed by the same body of common-law doctrines that governed traditional status hierarchies of parent–child, husband–wife, guardian–ward, master–servant, and master–apprentice. The subordinates in these relations (child, wife, ward, servant, apprentice) were defined as dependents who owed obedience and service to their superiors (father, husband, guardian, master). The superordinate in effect owned the labor of the subordinate and had the right to command obedience. Conversely, the superordinate had a reciprocal obligation to provide his subordinate with support and protection and, in the case of children and apprentices, with education or training.[4]

Regulation of labor relations and family relations by the same body of law perhaps made sense in the seventeenth and eighteenth centuries when both sets of relations usually took place in a common space, namely the household. However, over the course of the nineteenth century, home and market became increasingly separate domains both materially and ideologically. An economy based primarily on small producers—farmers, artisans, planters, laborers, mechanics, and small businessmen—was gradually transformed into one dominated by corporate ownership and wage labor. While the family/household remained the site of reproduction and caring, production increasingly took place in workplaces outside of the home. Changes in ideology accompanied these economic transformations. Family life and economic life came to be conceived as separate and distinct spheres—private and public—governed by different principles.[5]

In the years following the American Revolution, feudal traditions embodied in common law came to be seen as incompatible with a democratic polity. Whereas previously ownership of property had been the measure of independence required for suffrage and political participation, white journeymen and mechanics adopted the mantle of "free labor," claiming that ownership of their own labor and their freedom to contract gave them independence and therefore entitlement to full political rights. In the early decades of the nineteenth century most states did away with property requirements for voting and granted universal white manhood suffrage.[6]

Indentured servitude came to be viewed as inconsistent with the ideal of free labor and the status of white manhood. Up until the end of the eighteenth century it had been common for European immigrants to enter into indenture for a period of years in order to pay for their passage and establish themselves in a trade. By the third decade of the nineteenth century most states had passed laws banning indentured servitude whereby white workers could no longer bind themselves or be bound to fixed terms of employment as had been the case under master–servant acts.[7]

Free labor status was, however, limited to white men. The enslavement of African Americans continued until 1865, and indentured contract labor for Chinese and other immigrants of color continued into the late nineteenth century. Moreover, freedom of employment was curtailed by the exclusion of workers of color from many trades and from white-collar jobs. As a result, free blacks were restricted to a few occupations involving heavy physical labor or "dirty work." Whereas black men were concentrated in agricultural field labor or in "unskilled" labor and service jobs, black women were overwhelmingly concentrated in field labor or some branch of domestic service, including laundering. Because workers of color did not have many choices, employers could keep wages artificially low.[8]

Belated Feudalism

Early twentieth-century legal scholars looking back on the changes that had occurred in labor relations during the nineteenth century described them as representing an overall shift from status to contract.

Instead of rights and obligations being attached to one's status as master or servant, rights and obligations were established by explicit or implicit contracts freely entered into by two theoretically equal parties. In the view of these early scholars, the shift occurred because contractual relations were more congruent with the needs of modern commercial society, which rested on individualism and the capacity of individuals to contract their own labor.[9]

Late twentieth-century labor scholars challenged these interpretations, identifying what Karen Orren called "belated feudalism" surviving well into the twentieth century. According to these scholars, patriarchal principles embodied in common law were not eliminated but rather reconfigured in light of free-labor principles. Freedom of contract may have applied at the moment when the worker entered into employment, presumably by choice, but once employed the worker was bound by common-law tenets governing master–servant relationships. The employer retained the right to set (and change) the terms and conditions of employment—wages, hours, location and pace of work, timing of breaks, and required overtime. Employers could set rules that impinged on worker's lives off the job, for example, requiring them to live in company housing. In some industries, such as mining and forestry, it was common practice for the company to withhold workers' pay until the end of the contract period, forcing workers to rely on credit to pay for living expenses. This practice effectively bound workers to their jobs because they would have to immediately repay any debts they owed their employer when they left. In company towns, some employers paid workers in scrip that could be redeemed only at a company-owned store. Employers argued, and many courts agreed, that these practices were not inconsistent with a free labor system because workers retained the right to refuse a job or to quit it. Whether or not workers had the ability to actually exercise their theoretical rights in the real world was not at issue.[10]

Starting in the latter part of the nineteenth century, some state legislatures began to address the imbalance in power between employer and employee. They passed legislation requiring employers to pay wages weekly, to pay in cash or in scrip redeemable for cash, and to allow inspectors to check for honest weighing of coal output, upon which pay was based. During the Progressive Era, some states also passed statutes establishing maximum hours. However, before the mid-1930s courts, including the U.S. Supreme Court, regularly struck down state laws that set maximum hours for workers on the grounds that such laws infringed on liberty of contract. In their view, laws regulating hours, wages, and working conditions violated the due process clause of the Fourteenth Amendment to the Constitution, which guaranteed the right to make contract.

In its precedent-setting decision in Lochner v. New York (1905), the Supreme Court overturned a New York statute limiting the hours of bakers to 10 hours a day and 60 hours a week. The majority opinion stated that the statute "interfered with the right of contract between the employer and employe[e]s concerning the number of hours in which the latter may labor in the bakery of the employer." The Court further elaborated on freedom of contract in Coppage v. Kansas (1915), which overturned a Kansas Supreme Court decision upholding a state law forbidding employers making employment conditional on the worker signing an agreement to not be a member of the union. The Court specifically addressed the issue of the vastly unequal economic power of employer and employee that the Kansas Court had cited in its upholding of the statute. The Supreme Court averred that "inequalities of fortune" were an inevitable consequence of the right of private property but that the freedom of contract clause applied equally to employers and employees, regardless of inequalities of fortune.[11]

A major exception was made for laws regulating work hours for women. In this instance, defenders of the laws successfully argued that the government's interest in protecting women's procreative capacity outweighed preserving their freedom of contract. In 1908, the U.S. Supreme Court, in Muller v. Oregon, upheld an Oregon law that set a maximum of 10 hours a day for women working in laundries and factories.[12] Thus, ironically, women workers received the benefit of state protection precisely because they were considered to be weaker and therefore not fully "free and independent workers." They thus could not freely engage in contract.

Protective labor laws for women, however, were limited to those in specific industries; maximum-hour laws did not apply to domestic workers, even though their workdays were among the longest of all occupations. The lack of regulation of domestic and personal service workers particularly affected black women because they were overwhelmingly concentrated in these fields. According to the 1910 U.S.

Census, 853,302 black women were employed in domestic and personal services. The numbers reported fell to 780,592 in the 1920 Census but rose to 1,152,560 by 1930. In a study of black domestic workers conducted for the Women's Bureau of the U.S. Department of Labor, Jean Collier Brown reported that "The typical hours were 72 a week. There were 16 reports of 80 to 90 hours and there was one report of a week of 91 hours."[13]

Significantly, minimum-wage laws for women did not receive the same support as maximum-hour laws for women. Altogether 16 states passed minimum-wage laws for women between 1912 and the early 1920s. Most of these laws were invalidated by the Supreme Court. In 1923, in Adkins v. Children's Hospital, the Court struck down a Washington, D.C. minimum-wage law for women on the familiar grounds that it violated freedom of contract. The effect of placing a ceiling on women's work hours but no floor on their wages was to lower women's earning capacity.[14]

A New Deal, but not for Domestic Workers

Up until the 1930s the regulation of labor relations was left to the individual states for the most part. Only with the election of Franklin Delano Roosevelt as President in 1932 did the U.S. Congress begin to pass legislation that set national standards for wages, hours, unionization, and working conditions. In his inauguration speech, Roosevelt promised Depression-era Americans, especially the millions suffering from unemployment, a New Deal.[15] Within 100 days of his taking office, Roosevelt prevailed on Congress to pass several pieces of legislation to jump-start the economy.

The National Industrial Recovery Act (NIRA) of 1933 was one of the boldest. In addition to mandating an ambitious program of public works to increase employment, the NIRA offered concessions to both capital and labor. It lifted constraints on industrial cartels from anti-trust laws while it established workers' rights to join unions and unions' rights to bargain for industry-wide wages. It also required companies to write industry-wide codes of fair competition that established minimum wage levels and price floors. The drawing up of codes was overseen by the National Recovery Administration (NRA), a body created by executive order. Companies that signed on and stayed in compliance with the codes were allowed to display the NRA "Blue Eagle" as a symbol that "we do our part."[16]

The rationale for federal laws setting standards for labor contracts was Congress's constitutionally defined responsibility to regulate interstate commerce. However, the U.S. Supreme Court interpreted the interstate commerce clause narrowly to mean literally the movement of goods between states, and ruled the NIRA unconstitutional in May 1935.[17]

Although the NIRA did not survive, key features of it were incorporated into what are now considered landmark pieces of legislation that "modernized" labor relations. Section 7a[18] on workers' rights to form and join unions was incorporated into the National Labor Relations Act of 1935 (often called the Wagner Act for its principal Senate framer). The Wagner Act affirmed workers' rights to form and join unions, legalized their right to strike, and barred employers from firing them for engaging in union activities. Importantly, the Wagner Act established a federal agency, the National Labor Relations Board (NLRB), to investigate and adjudicate charges of unfair labor practices, arbitrate labor–management disputes, and oversee elections in which workers could decide on union representation.[19]

The Fair Labor Standards Act (FLSA), drafted by Secretary of Labor Frances Perkins, was introduced in 1937, following Roosevelt's landslide victory in 1936. It was finally enacted in 1938 after considerable struggle because of opposition from Southern Democrats. The FLSA established a federal minimum wage rate (initially 25 cents per hour), maximum hours (44 hours a week), and overtime provisions (time and a half) for many occupations. It also forbade the payment of wages in scrip unless that scrip was redeemable in cash.[20]

Both the NLRB and FLSA survived legal challenges. By the time of the passage of the NLRB and the FLSA, the U.S. Supreme Court had shifted from its earlier pattern of striking down state minimum-wage and other labor legislation—decisions that became highly unpopular in Depression Era America, even among conservatives. In 1936 Roosevelt had run on a platform that made national labor standards legislation a central feature of his campaign. His reelection by a landslide and his threat to pack the Supreme Court sent a strong message that the nation was crying out for change. For the first time, in March of 1937, the Court upheld a state minimum wage law, a Washington state statute setting minimum wages for women and children.[21] Two weeks later, on April 12, 1937, it upheld the constitutionality of the NLRB, and three years later in 1941, it upheld the FLSA.[22]

Some political scientists, such as Karen Orren and Richard A. Brisbin, date the establishment of "modern" employer–employee relations to the passage of these two pieces of landmark labor legislation.[23] Yet, if these laws can be said to have modernized labor relations, then domestic work remained "unmodernized."

The National Labor Relations Act

The NLRA specifically exempted "any individual employed . . . in the domestic service of any family or person at his home." It also exempted railroad and government workers (who received similar coverage under different statutes) and agricultural workers (who are sometimes covered under state laws). Thus, domestic workers employed in private homes were left as the only major low-level workers to be completely excluded from protection of their organizing rights.[24] The exemption was made despite the fact that there was a significant history of organizing by paid domestic workers prior to the passage of the NLRA. This history of organization belied the claim that it was impractical to organize workers in scattered worksites with multiple employers.[25] The exemption of domestic workers was not changed in major amendments to the Wagner Act in 1947 (Taft Hartley) and 1959 and 1974, and no alternative statute covers domestic workers, so they have remained excluded from organizing under the protection of labor laws until the present day.[26]

Analysis of court decisions and Congressional discussions about the exclusion of domestic service from laws regulating labor relations indicates that the ideology of separate spheres and the desire to maintain the family and household as a protected private sphere have profoundly shaped the view of paid caring labor as "not really work." By reason of its location in the home, paid caring labor has been treated by the legal system similarly to unpaid domestic labor, as a labor of love and thus not subject to market calculation. Courts have sometimes been explicit in citing the home as a site of intimate personal relations rather than a site of labor. In 1939, a Minnesota court upheld the conviction of a domestic worker for constituting a nuisance by picketing in front of the home of his employer on the grounds that the worker was not entitled to protection by a Minnesota statute entitling all workers the right to organize, saying the home "is a sacred palace for people to go and be quiet and at rest and not be bothered with the turmoil of industry."[27]

That the location of the work in the home and the supposed family nature of relations in that setting are the determinative factors in continuing to exclude domestic work from NLRA protection is confirmed by later NLRB decisions. For example, in a 1979 case the board distinguished between workers who perform domestic tasks for maid agencies, office and condominium complexes, and hotels, who were protected, and workers who are "in the domestic service of any family or persons at his home," who were not."[28]

The Fair Labor Standards Act

Similar considerations have operated in relation to FLSA, which also exempted domestic workers. Some exemptions, such as for agricultural workers, were made as a response to the wishes of specific economic interests. Service occupations in general were excluded on the assumption that these occupations lay within the realm of intrastate commerce and were subject only to state laws. Thus many low-paid women workers in restaurants, laundries, hotels, and hairdressing establishments were excluded from minimum-wage and maximum-hour standards. Domestic work also fit in this category, but additionally its exclusion was determined by being seen as belonging to a different sphere than other forms of labor. Historian Vivien Hart points out that Roosevelt himself reassured southerners who were concerned that the FLSA would require that housewives "pay your negro girl eleven dollars a week," stating: "No law ever suggested intended a minimum wages and hours bill to apply to domestic help." Hart points out "the fact that the President thought of these women as help, not as labor, sums up their problem."[29]

The version of the FLSA that was finally passed in 1938 was considerably watered down from earlier proposals, especially with regard to enforcement mechanisms. Some women workers in manufacturing benefited by having the same minimum wage as men; however, the vast majority of women workers were excluded from federal protection by virtue of being in retail sales and service occupations. Up until the

1970s, care workers in institutionalized settings as well as in private households—disproportionately black women—continued to be exempt not only from federal minimum-wage and maximum-hour standards but also from state laws that were often broader in their coverage.[30]

The "Companionship" Exemption

The civil rights movement and the women's movement of the 1960s and 1970s impelled a new focus on government employment policy by addressing discrimination against and denial of equal opportunity and equal protection to women and minority workers. The Equal Pay Act of 1963 mandated equal pay for equal work regardless of gender or race. This legislation, although symbolically important, had only limited impact. Segregation of the labor market by race and gender meant that men and women, whites and blacks, rarely held exactly the same jobs. Thus most wage inequality was a result of unequal pay scales for predominately male jobs and predominately female jobs.

Title VII of Civil Rights Act of 1964 was a more comprehensive fair employment law. It prohibited discrimination on the basis of sex, race, color, religion, and national origin and also called for affirmative action by employers to provide equal opportunity to groups that had suffered discrimination in the past.[31] The shift in climate in Washington and the nation was also reflected in renewed efforts to get the U.S. Congress to extend worker benefits and protections to groups that had heretofore been excluded from coverage.

In 1973, the Democratic-dominated Congress introduced bills in the Senate and House to amend the Fair Labor Standards Act in major ways. Among the proposed reforms was the lifting of the exemption of retail, service, and domestic workers. The inclusion of domestic workers was strongly supported by liberal northern Democrats, women, and black members of Congress. The proponents stressed the importance of conferring dignity and recognition to women who were doing work that was not accorded respect by members of society. As Representative Edith Green (D-OR) stated it, "Mr. Chairman, ultimately it seems to me the question must resolve itself into one of simple justice. Do we really want anyone in our society to work 40 hours a week and not earn an income at least approaching the poverty level?"[32] Other proponents cited studies documenting the dire situation of women domestics, the majority of whom were heads of households and many of whom were forced to supplement their meager earnings with welfare. Black congressmen and women proponents, such as Parren Mitchell (D-MD) and Shirley Chisolm (D-NY), spoke about the long history of discrimination that had forced black women into domestic service and attested to their own mothers' and grandmothers' experience of having to work as domestics.[33]

Proponents of covering domestic workers referred to the anomaly that the demand for domestic work was growing at the same time that the number of women working as domestics was dropping and argued that higher wages would reverse the trend. As Representative Mark Gaydos (D-PA) argued, "An increase in the minimum wage protections and the overtime provision of the act will very likely bring increased workers into the market place."[34] In arguing that extending minimum wage would make domestic work more attractive and thus increase the supply of household workers, Gaydos and other proponents portrayed domestic workers as rational economic actors.

The Republicans offered substitute bills in both the Senate and the House that would have eliminated the provision adding domestic workers to the occupations covered by FLSA. Republicans argued that the minimum-wage provision would be unenforceable because of the sheer numbers of employers and the inability of housewives to cope with the complicated paperwork. Representative John Erlenborn (R-IL), who had offered a substitute bill, opined about the majority bill: "I think the provision to extend coverage to domestic workers is one of the most mischievous in the bill. This will require every housewife who employs a worker on a 1-day-week basis or even a half-day a week basis to keep books and records as the time spent by that domestic worker." The minority report stated, "Do we really want to subject housewives to possible criminal penalties for failure to keep these records accurately? Can we expect enforcement?"[35]

What seemed to be at stake in the arguments were not just notions of social justice and dignity but cultural conceptions of the home and domestic labor.[36] Proponents of FLSA coverage for domestics, reflecting the rhetoric of the 1970s women's and civil rights movements, put forth a view of household work as skilled and valuable labor and thus deserving of adequate wages and protection from overwork. Representative Bertram L. Podell (D-NY), for example, stated:

We should admit once and for all that those persons who perform the tasks of domestic employment are providing a valuable economic product. Not only are they contributing to the economy, they are also making it possible for many others to make use of their talents outside the confines of the home. We should recognize the great contributions made by domestic workers by extending to them the coverage of a decent minimum age, as provided for in the bill before us.[37]

Representative Martha Griffith (D-MI) defended not only minimum wage for domestic workers but also a tax deduction for their employers:

What the gentleman really is saying is what that woman does in a home is of no worth. I should like to differ with him. What she does in that home is a thing that makes life livable. She is entitled to a decent wage, and her employer, whether it is a gentleman or his wife, is entitled to deduct that before he pays his taxes.[38]

Shirley Chisolm refuted some House members' objections that housewives lacked the business knowledge needed to maintain tax, social security, and other records for their domestic employees by stressing the competence needed to maintain a home, and, by implication, the skilled nature of household labor.

This may come as a shock to the Members of this House, but in most homes it is the wife who handles the family budget, and bookkeeping. She can tell you how much you owe at the bank, on the car loan, the charges run up on her credit cards, and in these days of spiraling food prices, she has been doing plenty of fancy figuring about base prices and unit prices in grocery stores. To suggest that women do not know how to add and subtract is an insult to women and totally contrary to all existing evidence.[39]

Not just women members of Congress but also some liberal male Democrats understood the relationship between the devaluation of unpaid housework and the low status of paid domestic service. Senator Harrison Arlington Williams Jr. (D-NJ) noted:

The lack of respect accorded domestics is in many ways an unfortunate reflection of the value we placd [sic] on the traditional role of women in our society.

The housewife's job has always been considered of secondary importance, even though it is the housewife who is entrusted with our most valuable resources and our most valuable material possession, our children and our home. In hiring a domestic, most employers expect her to accept many of the responsibilities of the homemaker thereby creating a situation in which a dollar value is being placed on her everyday duties.

Considering the current wage for domestics, it would mean that we are placing an $.80 an hour value on the work done by every housewife in America. This hardly seems reasonable."[40]

In contrast, opponents drew on images of the home as a place of repose and leisure and characterized household work as unskilled and undemanding. In the Senate, Republicans Peter Dominick (R-NM) and Robert Taft Jr. (R-OH) sponsored the Senate version of the minority bill that omitted domestic workers. Senator Dominick repeatedly referred to the hypothetical case of a 14-year-old neighbor boy who, hired to mow the lawn, would dawdle if he were being paid a minimum hourly wage. As for full-time domestic workers, Dominick imagined them enjoying long periods of leisure and thus not really working much of the time.

> What do we do about the cleaning lady that comes in? She enjoys herself. She gets together with the family and has a coke or a glass of milk. She has business with the family. She cleans up and does a good job. We pay her a living wage but she is doing a lot for other people as well as for me. She has got a regular business going. In most cases, she is being paid far more than the minimum wage if she happens to be a cleaning woman, because they are so very hard to get these days.[41]

He also read a letter from a constituent who employed a housekeeper as a caregiver for her mother while she herself worked as a secretary:

> Even if the salary is not $2 an hour—for the small amount of work required in my apartment, the leisure time spent there watching TV, reading, relaxing, visiting with my mother, using my telephone, eating me out of "house and home," plus the additional FICA tax I must pay quarterly, I consider that my domestic has a "good deal" going for her. Where can I get a job that gives me all these "extras" that are tax-free and not included in my salary? [42]

In contrast to Democratic proponents who assumed that domestic workers were rational economic actors, who would respond to higher pay and better working conditions by entering or staying in domestic service, Republican opponents emphasized the familial qualities of domestic work relations and evoked the traditional image of household workers as faithful family retainers. Thus their Minority Report opined that should minimum wage standards be imposed, "retired individuals and social companions who might perform infrequent tasks for a household may have to be asked to leave for economic reasons. It certainly is a sorry state of affairs when the Government forces such lifelong, loyal employees and friends from households in their senior years."[43] Other opponents drew on conceptions of African Americans as incapable and unproductive and therefore likely to be fired if their employers had to pay them a minimum wage. Senator Taft predicted that rather than paying higher wages to an inefficient employee, a housewife "would use an increased number of electrical appliances and machines."[44]

The substitute bill was defeated, but when the final version of the bill came up for a vote, it included significant compromises. It included only domestic workers who worked at least 8 hours a week or whose earnings over the year were high enough to require deductions for Social Security. It specifically exempted from minimum wage and overtime provisions "employees employed on a casual basis in domestic service employment to provide babysitting services" and domestic service employees employed "to provide companionship services for individuals who (because of age or infirmity) are unable to care for themselves." It also exempted from the overtime provision "domestic service employees who reside in the household in which they are employed."[45]

The exemption of live-in domestics from maximum hours was based on a committee report that stated: "Ordinarily such an employee engages in normal private pursuits such as eating, sleeping, and entertaining, and has other periods of complete freedom. In such a case it would be difficult to determine the exact hours worked."[46] In discussing the companionship exemption, Democratic members of Congress adopted the Republicans' template of companionship services as being the kind of work done by a teenager or neighbor who came in occasionally for a few hours to baby sit; they then applied that template to the services of full-time childcare and home elder care providers. An exchange between Senators Quentin Burdick (D-ND) and Harrison Williams (D-NJ), both supporters of the Democratic bill, is instructive.

Senator Burdick had drawn the attention of his colleagues to the fact that the committee's report was not intended to include "domestic service such activities as babysitting and acting as a companion." He observed that these categories referred to two scenarios: "We have situations of young people, a widow, a divorcee, or a family of low income, which of necessity must have someone sit with their children while they are at work," and "people who might have an aged father, an aged mother, an infirm father, an infirm mother, and a neighbor comes in and sits with them." Senator Burdick concluded, "This, of course, entails some work, such as perhaps making lunch for the children or making lunch for the infirm person, and may even require throwing some diapers in the automatic washing machine for the baby. This would be incidental to the main purpose of the employment."[47]

Senator Williams clarified the meaning of companion to mean "the situation in which people are in a household not to do household work but are there, first, as babysitters. I think we all have the full meaning of what a babysitter is there for—to watch the youngsters." This quick exchange then occurred:

> *Mr. Burdick:* "Companion," as we mean it, is in the same role—to be there and to watch an older person, in a sense.
> *Mr. Burdick:* In other words, an elder sitter.
> *Mr. Williams:* Exactly.[48]

The Amendment to the FLSA finally passed both houses of Congress and was signed into law by President Richard M. Nixon on April 8, 1974.[49] Unfortunately, the law as passed contained a few "poison-pill" characteristics, most notably the "companionship exemption."

It appears obvious, from reading the records of Congressional debates on the FSLA provisions on domestic service, babysitting, and companionship service, that members of Congress were focused only on situations in which housewives, parents of children, and children of frail elderly persons employed baby sitters and elder care givers in their own homes. However, in promulgating regulations based on the new legislation, the Division on Wages and Hours of the Department of Labor (DOL) interpreted the "companionship" exemption to cover a much larger group of workers than Congress had intended.

First, the DOL interpreted the term "private home" broadly to include caregivers working in assisted living facilities and other congregate housing. When workers mounted legal challenges to the DOL position, courts came up with complex criteria by which to arrive at a determination on a case-by-case basis. Such factors as the source of funding, degree of access to the facility by the general public, profit or non-profit status, and the size of the sponsoring organization were taken into account in order to decide whether a particular residence was more similar to a home or to an institution or business.[50]

The DOL also broadened exemptions to legislative requirements by expanding the kinds of tasks that could be counted as part of "companionship services." The DOL regulations interpreted "companionship services" to refer to day-to-day care of elderly or infirm individuals and limited the amount of "general housework" to 20 percent of the total weekly hours worked. However, much of what would normally be thought of as "housework" is included in the DOL's definition of companionship services. According to DOL regulations, companionship services could include any amount of "household work related to the care of the aged or infirm person such as meal preparation, bed making, washing of clothes or similar services."[51]

Most importantly, the DOL exempted from FLSA protection not only caregivers employed by disabled or frail elderly persons or by their families but also home health aides and certified nursing assistants employed by private agencies and supervised by registered nurses. In none of the Congressional debates on companionship services was there any reference to workers employed by non-profit agencies or profit-making companies that assigned them to care for frail elderly clients. Because agency workers had been covered prior to the 1974 amendments to the FLSA, home-care workers actually lost coverage under the reforms that were supposedly designed to extend protection to those previously excluded.

The DOL interpretation of "companionship services" has been continuously criticized by home-care workers, unions, and public interest groups. In 2001, the Secretary of Labor issued a memo announcing that the Department was proposing to remove the lack of protection for caregivers employed by agencies, but after a period of public comment, the DOL quietly withdrew the proposal in 2002. Powerful interests were vested in continuing the exclusion: both profit-making agencies wanting to maximize profit and state agencies seeking to contain costs consistently opposed extending FLSA protection to agency-employed home-care workers. Unions representing home-care workers and organizations dedicated to the interests of recipients of care, such as AARP (the organization formerly known as the American Association of Retired Persons) and the Independent Living Movement, lobbied for inclusion on the grounds that providing better wages and working conditions would attract higher quality workers and decrease turnover, but they have had less political clout than the opponents of covering home care workers.[52]

Returning now to the case of Evelyn Coke v. Long Island Care at Home, Ltd. with which we began the chapter, we can see the opposing interests represented in the prolonged court battle waged over the DOL's decision to exempt companies employing home care workers from FLSA coverage. With legal support from the Service Employees International Union (SEIU), Coke filed a lawsuit against the company that employed her, Long Island Care at Home, Ltd., challenging the DOL regulations and claiming back wages owed her from unpaid overtime. Her attorneys argued that the DOL's position was inconsistent with legislative intent and with other federal regulations. Amicus curiae briefs supporting Coke were filed by AARP, Older Women's League, Alliance for Retired Americans, American Association of People with Disabilities, National Women's Law Center, and the American Civil Liberties Union; conversely briefs supporting Long Island Care at Home, Ltd. were filed by the New York State Association of Health Care Providers, Continuing Care Leadership Coalition, Inc., the Corporation Counsel of the City of New York, and the U.S. Secretary of Labor.[53]

In 2003, the U.S. Federal Appeals Court for the Second District had ruled that the DOL regulations were merely interpretations and thus did not have the force of law. The court also found that the exemption of employees of for-profit and non-profit agencies from FLSA coverage conflicted with other regulations and that there were gaps in the DOL's reasoning. The DOL immediately issued a memo detailing its rationale for exemption and an advisory letter stating that, the federal court ruling notwithstanding, the exemption could be assumed to hold in all other jurisdictions. On appeal in 2004, the U.S. Supreme Court remanded the case back for reconsideration by the Federal Appeals Court in light of a new DOL memorandum detailing its rationale for the exemption. The Federal Appeals Court reconsidered the Coke case and held in August 2006 that it found "no reason to abandon the reasoning or results reached" in its earlier ruling.[54]

In January 2007 the U.S. Supreme Court issued a writ of certiorari to the Federal Appeals Court (demanding its records of the case), and in April 2007 held a rehearing of the case. The main argument of counsel for Coke was that in passing the 1974 amendments to the Fair Labor Standards Act Congress was intending to broaden, not narrow, coverage. The justices for the most part focused on the technical matter of whether the DOL regulations were merely advisory or had the authority of law. Justice Ruth Bader Ginsberg expressed puzzlement that amendments that were intended to broaden coverage had in this case narrowed it. However, she did not draw any further implications or conclusions from the apparent contradiction created by the DOL regulations. The only justice who expressed concern about the real-life consequences of the case was Justice Breyer, who voiced concern primarily about families being unable to afford care for loved ones, so that millions of sick people would end up in institutions.[55] By focusing only on the entitlement of recipients to receive around-the-clock care, Breyer subordinated the needs and rights of those who actually performed the around-the-clock caring. On July 11, 2007, the Supreme Court issued a unanimous ruling that the DOL regulations were legally binding and therefore that home-care workers employed by companies were not entitled to minimum wage or overtime pay under the FLSA.[56] With this ruling the Court decreed that the burden of providing "affordable care" for vulnerable members of society would continue to be borne not by state or federal governments or corporations but by the poorest and most disadvantaged members of the work force.

Moreover, by failing to recognize any limitations on hours, the court reaffirmed the status of the domestic employee as property and of employers' entitlement to the services of the domestic employee as a property right. In her account of Progressive Era women reformers' efforts to convince middle-class women employers to modernize relationships with their employees by adopting voluntary limitations on work hours, Peggie Smith noted considerable resistance on the part of employers to any form of regulation:

> The typical household employer reasoned that as long as she had a domestic in her employ, she was *entitled* to expect around-the-clock service. Of course as a free laborer, the domestic could always terminate the relationship. While the relationship was in effect, though, the

prevailing sentiment held that she should be at virtually all times, accessible to the employer. Her very person belonged to the family for the duration of the employment arrangement, and thus, the family claimed a quasi-property right—couched in the language of family privacy—to exploit her labor without interference from government or imposition of a self-regulatory standard.

This reasoning, Smith asserts, amounted to the claim of a quasi-property right.[57]

Domestic Workers as Hired Property

The treatment of the employer–employee relationship in domestic service and home care as both a family-based status relationship and as a property relationship is starkly revealed by provisions in current immigration law. Classified as unskilled workers, domestic workers fall into the lowest preference category of those eligible for entry with green cards. Thus domestic workers have almost no chance of entering the United States as independent legal immigrants.

Contrarily, it is relatively easy for domestics to enter the United States as adjuncts or dependents of other high-priority immigrants, as B-1 visa holders. The federal government allows U.S. citizens returning temporarily after being abroad, and most non-immigrant visa holders, to bring dependents, which includes not only spouses and non-adult children but also "domestic or personal servants." Non-immigrant visa holders include those who enter the United States as foreign business travelers, entrepreneurs and investors, athletes and entertainers, religious workers, and/or those admitted for having special skills or being employed in special occupations. These B-1 visa-holding domestic employees can remain in the United States legally only as long as they remain employed by the primary visa holder.

The U.S. Citizenship and Immigration Services' main focus is on preventing fraudulent entry by those who are not genuine servants; by comparison there is little attention to protecting domestic employees once they are admitted. The primary visa holders are required to provide proof that the applicant servant is not abandoning his or her residence abroad and that he or she has had at least one year of experience as a servant, either for the visa holder or for someone else, prior to the application. However, according to Human Rights Watch, domestic workers who enter with B-1 visas are not entered on any Immigration Service database, so there is no registry of B-1 domestic workers, and the U.S. government does not know how many B-1 visas are issued each year. As a result, domestic workers entering under B-1 visas become invisible and unaccounted for.[58]

Additionally, the United States issues two other kinds of special visas for servants. Persons employed by diplomats and foreign consular officials and employees enter the country under A-3 visas, and those employed by officials and employees of international organizations such as the United Nations, the World Bank, and many others, enter under G-5 visas. Domestic positions that qualify for a G-5 visa include cooks, butlers, valets, maids, housekeepers, governesses, janitors, laundresses, caretakers, handymen, gardeners, grooms, chauffeurs, baby sitters, and companions to the aged or infirm.[59] The assumption behind both A-3 and G-5 visas is that the domestic or personal servant is a "dependent" of the principal visa holder. Thus, a holder of an A-3 or G-5 visa supposedly can remain in the United States only as long as she or he continues to work for the same employer and the employer remains in the United States.[60]

Employers of A-3 and G-5 visa holders are required to submit written contracts that set out conditions of employment: hours of work, medical insurance, compensation at the state or federal minimum wage or prevailing rate (whichever is greater), medical insurance, an agreement by the employer not to withhold the worker's passport, and agreement by the employee that she or he will not accept other employment while working for the principal visa holder. These provisions have been promulgated because of reported incidents of abuse and exploitation. However, there is no follow-up or monitoring by any of the agencies that are responsible for immigrants and/or workers, namely the U.S. State Department, Citizenship and Immigration Services, or the Labor Department. Human Rights Watch notes that no government agency or department keeps records of the contracts. Thus, there is no effort to verify employer compliance with the written contracts.[61]

Issues of exploitation of immigrant domestic workers will be discussed in greater detail in the next chapter. Here the focus has been on how immigration law treats domestic workers as dependents and quasi-family members rather than as independent immigrants. It is difficult to imagine that any other category of employees would be treated as dependents of other immigrants.

Conclusions

Despite the increased commodification of in-home caring labor and reliance on paid caregivers, paid caring has not been included in the "modernization" of labor relations. It has continued to be treated as part of the private family realm rather than as part of the market. As capitalist relations have penetrated more and more into social relations, there seems to be an even greater desire to preserve the distinction between home and market and to maintain the home as a private refuge from market values. By virtue of its location in the home, caring work, whether paid or unpaid, is treated as though it is governed by altruism and status obligations. As a result, paid domestic workers suffer various forms of exclusion from benefits and rights accorded other paid workers. Instead, like family members performing unpaid care, they are treated as dependents rather than true workers. Paid domestic workers suffer a similar exclusion of their labor from social citizenship and entitlements.

The exclusion of home-care workers from social citizenship rights stems not just from their enclosure within the private household and their "quasi-family" standing. Their exclusion also grows out of their status as "quasi-property." Like property, servants and other paid carers can be discarded when no longer useful. Unlike a family member, the home-care worker is not owed the kind of reciprocity that is due a family member, and the employer does not incur the kinds of obligations that are incurred toward family members who provide services. In this sense, paid caring labor done in the household is doubly coercive: it is part of the household system that is hierarchically organized according to common-law principles, and it is part of a property relationship that denies the independent personhood of the worker and vests property rights in the employer.

The exclusion from protections such as minimum wage and overtime requirements, occupational health and safety standards, unemployment insurance, workmen's compensation, and anti-discrimination law contributes to the poverty of home-care workers. Despite the great demand for their services, home-care workers are low paid, overworked, and lack health care themselves. Turnover is high because only those who lack other options and/or become attached to those they care for continue to work in home care for extended periods. Those who do persist are vulnerable to physical problems from repetitious lifting and straining. When they grow old, like Evelyn Coke, they find themselves poor, sick, without health coverage, and unprotected by legal safeguards granted to virtually all other workers in the country.

This is not the end of the story. Home-care workers have not pinned all of their hopes on court decisions or revisions of federal interpretations of FLSA. They have simultaneously worked to exert political and moral pressure on state, county, and city governments to pass bills mandating minimum wage, overtime, and other protections for home-care workers. In 2003, at the instigation of domestic worker organizations, the New York City Council passed a bill requiring placement agencies to obtain signed promises from employers to follow minimum wage, overtime, and Social Security regulations. In 2008 CASA de Maryland won a bill to require employers in Montgomery County, Maryland, to provide employees with written contracts setting out wages and benefits.[62] In a closely watched campaign, a Domestic Workers' Bill of Rights (DWBR), covering housekeepers, nannies, and eldercare workers, wended its way through the New York State legislature in 2009. The key provisions of the bill provided for "a limited number of paid sick days, personal days, and vacation days; notice and severance pay; yearly raises tied to inflation; full overtime pay for any work over 40 hours per week; one day of rest per week; protection from employment discrimination; and health benefits."[63] An earlier, less comprehensive bill was passed by the California legislature in 2006 but was vetoed by Republican governor Arnold Schwarzenegger. Subsequently the California Coalition for Household Worker Rights announced that it would be working to pass a domestic worker rights bill through the California legislature in 2010.[64]

With the election of Barack Obama and sizable Democratic majorities in the Senate and House in the 2008 federal elections, Evelyn Coke's fight was renewed at the federal level. On June 15, 2009, 15 U.S. senators and 37 members of the House of Representatives wrote a letter to Secretary of Labor Hilda Solis asking her to end the exclusion of in-home workers from coverage by the Fair Labor Standards Act. They wrote, "Evelyn Coke, who took a case all the way to the Supreme Court, spent two decades working more than 40 hours a week caring for others. Yet, when she suffered from kidney failure, she could not afford a health care worker to take care of her." Secretary Solis responded positively, promising to "fulfill the department's mandate to protect America's workers, including home health care aides, who work demanding schedules and receive low wages." Less than a month later, on July 9, 2009, Evelyn Coke passed away in Manhasset, New York. Her son Michael Findley said that he thought "a serious bedsore had contributed to her death, and recalled the many people she had helped with bedsores."[65]

6

Neoliberalism and Globalization

Demographic and cultural changes, neoliberal economic policies, and economic globalization are among the contemporary developments exacerbating the care crisis by intensifying the conflicts between caring and earning and increasing the stresses on caregivers, both unpaid and paid. Numerous studies have documented the tremendous growth in the population of disabled children and adults and elderly persons in industrialized countries. In the United States, because of federal and state health and disability policies favoring home-based care, a substantial majority of those needing long-term care live at home rather than in institutional settings. The U.S. Department of Health and Human Services, using 2000 Census data, estimated that 13 million Americans with disabilities, including children and working-age adults, were living in private homes; it also projected that this number will more than double by 2050, with much of the increase coming from a rise in the elderly population.[1]

At the same time that the population of those needing home-based care has been expanding, the capacity of informal care givers—families and friends—to provide care has been shrinking. Demographically, the working-age population aged 18–64 is growing much more slowly than the population 65 years and older.[2] Social changes such as smaller family size, geographic mobility, and the increase in full-time employment among women are reducing the number and availability of family members and friends who can provide unpaid caring labor.[3]

Because they have fewer people with whom they can share the load, those who do provide informal care are more burdened. Employed women who also perform caring tasks are stretched by the competing demands of earning and care. Rates of poverty, drug dependency, and incarceration have also increased such that many parents are unable to care for their children. As a result, more distant relatives may assume responsibility for children to avoid having them sent into foster care. Indeed, one of the most notable trends over the past two decades has been the increasing numbers of grandparents, and even great grandparents— mostly women—who are the primary caretakers of children. Some of these grandmothers may also have their own elderly parents and relatives to care for and have their own health problems that make caring difficult.[4]

Perhaps most fundamental are economic changes brought about by so-called neoliberal economic policies and globalization. The shifting of production outside the United States has reduced the number and percentage of relatively well-paying unionized manufacturing jobs. The growing service and retail sectors offer primarily low-wage, part-time, and contingent employment, usually without benefits. Simultaneously, under neoliberal restructuring, government spending on welfare entitlements has been cut, and public services have been subcontracted to private companies. In the meantime, neoliberal policies have been imposed by international banking and financial institutions on developing countries. These policies have included the selling off of state enterprises to private entities, the appropriation of land formerly used for subsistence agriculture to produce large-scale export crops, and the opening of formerly protected markets to foreign products. These measures have left millions of people in developing countries without their traditional means of livelihood. As a consequence, many people have turned to migration to find work in more prosperous areas. Significant portions of migrants, especially women, find jobs in low-wage service sectors in the global north.

These developments have had multifarious consequences for caring labor. Rather than dealing with the many and complex ramifications of these developments, I will focus on three representative case studies that typify trends in the present period: health care cost containment that has led to the "off-loading" of health care to family caregivers; welfare reform that has diverted poor women's labor from family care to low-wage employment; and the deinstitutionalization and privatization of care for the elderly disabled that has further disadvantaged home-care workers.

Intensifying Home Care

One of most noteworthy trends in recent decades has been the off-loading of medical treatment for both acute and chronic conditions from hospital to homes. This shifting is part of a larger strategy within the service sector to transfer work from paid employees to consumers, thereby reducing labor costs and maximizing profits. Examples of work transfer include replacing counter clerks and sales people with customer self-service in retail trade, replacing tellers with automated teller machines in banking, and replacing reservation clerks with on-line booking in the airline industry.[5]

In the medical arena, work transfer has been driven by cost-containment structures imposed by health-care delivery and health-care financing systems. Pressure to slash health-care costs by insurance companies and some government agencies has resulted in the shortening of costly hospital stays. Patients are released to go home "quicker and sicker" while they still require medical monitoring and nursing care. Additionally, the deinstitutionalization and independent living movements have supported the shift toward home-based care. Politically organized disabled persons have lobbied to get laws passed requiring states to provide services and accommodations that will to allow them to live independently in their communities.

The ideological rationale for deinstitutionalization is that the home offers a superior environment for the patient. It draws on stereotypes of home and hospital as starkly different. As William Ruddick notes, "Home is commonly conceived and experienced as a place of security, comfort, privacy, and liberty to be oneself. By contrast the hospital is often thought of and experienced as a place of insecurity, discomfort, intrusion, and demands for compliance and conformity.[6] The economic rationale for deinstitutionalized care is that extended hospital and nursing-home care is too costly and should be reserved for short-term treatment until the patient is "stabilized." The lower cost of home and community care is premised on the assumption that all or most of the care will be provided for free by family members and volunteers.

Thus, since the 1970s there has been a general trend away from institutional care for chronically ill or disabled children and adults and frail elderly. The consequence is that more people are being cared for at home, and more people are providing more unpaid caring for relatives, neighbors, and friends. A *New York Times* article in 1999 reported that an estimated 26 million Americans were providing nursing services such as administering medication and checking vital signs for sick or dependent relatives, putting in an average of 18 hours per week. A survey by the National Caregiver Alliance and AARP (the organization formerly known as the American Association of Retired Persons) published in 2004 found that 21 percent of adults were caring for relatives or friends 18 years of age or older.[7]

The contemporary transfer of care from the hospital to the home represents a reversal of the post–World War II expansion of institutionalized health care. In that period, the medical establishment succeeded in portraying the hospital as a superior environment for patient care because the home could not be kept sufficiently sterile and lacked the facilities and equipment to provide modern medical diagnosis and treatment. Physicians for the most part stopped making home visits. Instead, patients were expected to travel to or be transported to hospitals or clinics for diagnosis and treatment. In one sense, it would seem we have come full circle to an earlier period when the sick, disabled, and elderly were nursed at home by a female relative, neighbor, or friend. However, the rise of managed care, the bureaucratization of health financing, and the development of high-tech medical devices for home use have dramatically altered the demands of home care.

First, patients being released home today are on average sicker than in previous years and are often dependent on ventilators or other devices. They need more attention and for longer periods than those nursed at home in the past. Many would have died sooner from their underlying conditions in the past but are now kept alive much longer by modern drugs and high-tech medical devices. Starting in the 1980s, medical manufacturers entered the growing home health care field by developing and marketing portable, so-called user-friendly versions of high-tech medical devices for use in the home. High-tech devices designed for use by patients themselves and untrained family members include equipment for infusion therapy (administering anti-pain, antibiotic, antiviral, and chemotherapy medications through a vein); feeding tubes (parenteral and enteral infusion of nutrient solutions for those unable to process or absorb food); ventilators (delivering oxygen and suctioning mucus for those with cardiopulmonary disease); dialysis machines (removing waste and excess fluid for those with kidney disease); and monitoring systems (for apnea and cardiac functioning).[8]

Nancy Guberman and colleagues find it significant that "medical professionals have delegated highly complex medical and nursing activities, activities which they refuse to delegate to other semi-professional groups (nurse aides, home-care workers, etc.), to untrained family members." The willingness of medical professionals to delegate responsibility to family members signals that they are trivializing the demands of high-tech care.[9] The assumption seems to be that high-tech equipment makes specialized knowledge and skill unnecessary much in the way that the assembly line reduced reliance on workers' skill.

What is especially striking about high-tech home treatment is that the usual medical hierarchy in which physicians (at least theoretically) oversee the work of nurses and other hospital personnel does not operate. Indeed, physicians are notably absent. They don't follow up with patients, never observe treatment being given, and exercise no oversight. Once patients are released from the hospital or nursing home, they are on their own after a brief prerelease orientation and perhaps a few home visits by a nurse or technologist.

High-technology home medical devices have been touted (by manufacturers and health administrators) for giving patients greater autonomy and mobility, so that they can "sustain normal activities far from the hospital." In practice, the devices impose considerable restrictions. In a study that compared instruction manuals for equipment with the actual experience of patients and their family caregivers, Lehoux, Saint-Arnaud, and Richard found that "the devices always both enabled and constrained the patients' daily activities and broader lives." They reported, "Some patients compared their situation to patients worse off than themselves (lateral comparisons) and tended to define their technology as capacity enhancing. Others compared their current situation to their life before technology (historical comparisons) and were much more critical of restrictions imposed by technology." Indeed, some users of high-technology devices felt a kind of "slavery to technology." They might be able to go out to a social event, for example, but "the constant presence of supplies, such as syringes, masks and bandages, nonetheless reminds everyone around of the medical nature of the technology. Tubes and noises are obvious markers that something is wrong with the user. For instance, in the case of oxygen therapy . . . [the] device makes a regular schlock . . . schlick sound that is loud enough to be heard by people within a 2-metre range."[10]

There is a certain irony in the notion that users of high-tech home devices can live in the comfort of their own homes rather than in a sterile hospital environment. In practice, high-tech treatment transforms the home into a hospital-like setting. Space in the home has to be reconfigured to accommodate equipment, cords, tubes, and bulky supplies. In the case of oxygen therapy, the sound of the respirator is a constant background noise. Alice, a caregiver interviewed by Cameron Macdonald, described sleeping next to her ventilator-dependent husband as "sleeping with the living lung." Caregivers have to strive constantly to maintain an aseptic environment.[11]

Family dynamics and interpersonal relations are also affected by the imposition of new and often unwelcome roles and responsibilities. Patients may feel guilty for being burdens, and family caregivers may feel they have little choice but to accept the burden in order to save a loved one's life. Family schedules are dominated by the necessary routines of high-tech care—changing IVs, sterilizing equipment, and keeping track of supplies. Safety features that warn about possible malfunctions create a pervasive sense of anxiety for both care receivers and caregivers. Emergencies and technological "incidents" require immediate response. Macdonald notes that sometimes school-age children must learn to deal with machinery and provide care, as in the case of Suzanne's children, aged 16, 14, and 7. Suzanne's husband, Bill, was dependent on a ventilator, and Suzanne had to work full-time to support the entire family. Her children knew "how to recognize the meanings of different warning beeps from the ventilator, how to assist with kinked tubes, and how to help their father clear fluid from the tracheotomy site." Still, Suzanne worried: "Yeah my biggest fear is that some day one of the kids is going to walk in and find him on the floor. That just scares the living daylights out of me."[12] In these scenarios, the home as hospital is far from being the place of refuge and relaxation depicted in idealized conceptions of home.

The issue of coercion is highly germane to the circumstances of family members involved in high-tech home care. Possibilities for coercion arise in at least four ways: the degree to which individuals in particular status positions feel compelled to take on a disproportionate amount of high-tech care, the lack of alternatives (or only negative ones) for individuals making decisions about technology-dependent relatives, the extent to which individuals providing intensive high-tech home care lose aspects of their identities and personhood, and the difficulty of "opting out" either temporarily or permanently once an individual or family has assumed responsibility for home care.

Regarding the pressure of expectations, feminist historians such as Emily Abel have noted that the closest female relative is viewed as the natural choice to provide care.[13] Nel Noddings notes, "Traditionally, the only acceptable excuse a woman has been able to offer is competing duties to care. Thus, a woman with several small children might be able to suggest, without guilt or shame, that her unmarried sister accept the duty to care for their elderly parents. The unmarried sister, however, could not escape the duty to care by pointing to her own projects personal or professional."[14] Similarly, a parent, especially a mother, if offered the option of caring for a ventilator-dependent child at home rather than have the child cared for in an institution surely feels obligated to accept the burdens of home care; to do otherwise would be viewed by others as evidence of an unnatural lack of motherly instincts. To a lesser but still significant degree, spouses feel duty bound to care for a ventilator- or dialysis-dependent partner at home rather than having them stay in a nursing home; refusal would indicate a lack of commitment, with particularly harsh judgments placed on a wife for failing to do her spousal duty.

The latter examples raise a second aspect of coercion, which is the degree to which individuals actually have choice, namely acceptable alternatives from which to choose. Often the alternative to assuming complete responsibility for home care is placing the relative in a nursing home. Cameron Macdonald describes the situation of Veronica, a 50-year-old secretary who was caring for her father, who had end-stage emphysema. Although she was willing to care for him in her time off because she considered the available nursing home "ghastly," she resisted learning to suction his lungs when they filled with fluid. Instead she called 911 several times a week to have her father taken to the emergency room to get his lungs suctioned. Macdonald concludes, "At the time of our interview, she was receiving increased pressure on all sides to either learn the procedure or put him in a Medicaid-funded nursing home that she described as 'filthy and depressing.'"[15]

Sometimes the alternative is even direr, namely that the patient would be allowed to die. Macdonald reports on the case of Tina, a 40-year-old high school teacher whose brother needed a bone marrow transplant to treat his leukemia and would require 24-hour care after the transplant. Tina explained:

> The hospital social worker kept asking me if I could quit my job. Or if I could pay for a nurse to come in 24–7. She said he would need me to keep the house sanitary and that he couldn't be left alone for more than 20 minutes in case he spiked a fever and died. . . . Well I couldn't quit my job. I'm the only income and the only insurance for my kids. I asked her what would happen if I said no. She said he would be denied the procedure, even though his insurance would pay for it. Basically, he would die if I didn't find some way to get him 24-hour care. I couldn't believe it.

In the end Tina was able to line up 30 friends and relatives to take turns monitoring her brother's condition.[16]

A third issue that pertains to coercion is the degree to which caregivers surrender certain aspects of their personhood, such as violating valued aspects of their identity and giving up their own projects. For example, a mother of a technology-dependent child may have to administer procedures that inflict serious pain and suffering, thus violating a deeply valued self-identity as a protective mother who shields her child from pain and suffering.[17] She will also have to forego employment and activities that are important to her sense of self.

All caregivers who are enmeshed in full-time care find their autonomy restricted as their schedules are dictated by the needs of the care receiver, with little time to dedicate to their own pursuits. High-tech care is notable for exacerbating the loss of self because of the intensity and constancy of demands. By definition, a technology-dependent care receiver cannot survive if oxygen or fluids run out or equipment malfunctions. Thus the caregiver has to remain in close proximity to monitor conditions and to respond to alerts and emergencies. In such situations caregivers themselves are tethered to the demands of medical devices and confined to the home. One carer of an IV-dependent husband curtailed social activities, saying, "I didn't dare go out, absolutely not," and a wife responsible for performing dialysis four times a week said, "It's like being in jail, you can't go anywhere."[18] Another caregiver expressed the weight of accountability that was transferred along with the burden of care: "It's a huge responsibility. You think, what if something were to happen and you don't know what to do. Who's going to live with that on the conscience for the rest of their life. Not the hospital. Not the nurse. Not the guy with the pencils trying to save money. It's the person who will have had to live through that."[19]

Finally, there is the issue of whether and how high-tech carers can discontinue caring if they decide they no longer want to carry on. One of the main features of "free labor" is the right to leave a job; thus, being bound to work for an indefinite term is the essence of coercion. At present, not only are there no clearly defined limits to the burden that an individual or family group can be expected to take on, there are no clearly accepted means of exit for those who no longer want to continue caring. Families differ in their financial, physical, and emotional resources and therefore also differ in their capacity to provide care. Moreover, individual and family resources change over time and become eroded or even exhausted.

James Arras and Nancy Dubler argue that in a just society it would be understood that there are moral limits to what might reasonably be expected from caregivers. The notion of moral limits means not only that individuals and families not be pressured or made to feel guilty for refusing to take on what they see as an unsupportable burden. It also means that family members and friends who have taken on high-tech care have the right to change their minds if they find the burden unsupportable. Any arrangements thus need to be seen as provisional or for a specified contractual period and as requiring periodic reassessment.[20] Yet treating care arrangements as contingent and contractual would violate deeply held assumptions about family and home. What is supposed to distinguish the family from other institutions is that the love (caring) and dedication among members is unconditional and absolute. As Robert Frost wrote in his poem, "The Death of the Hired Man," "Home is the place where, when you have to go there, / They have to take you in."[21]

An underlying issue is that although managed care policies often focus on the welfare of the care receiver, they fail to take the welfare of unpaid caregivers into account.[22] Even studies on the impacts of high-technology home care, for example, tend to focus on the impacts on the health and well-being of the patient; relatively few studies have focused on the effects of providing high-tech care on family caregivers. This is another instance where focusing on the needs and welfare of care recipients can render caregivers and their labor invisible.

Devaluing Mother Care

Responsibility for caring labor in the home, whether for children, the elderly, or the disabled, has traditionally been defined as women's responsibility. In the case of single mothers who lacked support from a male breadwinner, this responsibility has always been problematic. As will be discussed below, local and federal assistance to poor single mothers has always been stingy, with the majority being disqualified on moral or racial grounds.

Yet, for a brief period from the 1960s to the 1980s struggles waged by civil rights activists created a climate that led the U.S. Congress to expand welfare so as to provide some semblance of a safety net for more single mothers and their children under Aid to Families with Dependent Children (AFDC). For the first time, sizable numbers of poor African American mothers were able to gain access to welfare. Even though whites still constituted the majority of AFDC recipients, the typical welfare recipient came to be viewed by the larger society as a single African American woman. Attacks on welfare intensified in the 1980s, feeding on historic racial prejudices. Influential critics such as Charles Murray and Lawrence Mead framed the issue as one of AFDC fostering "welfare dependency" and discouraging poor women from becoming self-sufficient through employment.[23] Thus, simultaneously with medical cost-containment policies that have forced family members to take on more unpaid care work for sick and disabled relatives living at home, so-called welfare reform has sought to reduce spending on income support by diverting poor single mothers' labor from caring for their own children into paid employment outside the home. Reform efforts culminated in the enactment of the Personal Responsibility and Work Opportunity Reconciliation Act of 1996, which abolished AFDC and replaced it with Temporary Aid to Needy Families (TANF). TANF was designed to end welfare as an entitlement, limiting welfare benefits to five years over one's lifetime and making benefits contingent on efforts to get paid work. It also devolved responsibility for policy making and administrative oversight from the federal government to state and local entities and to the private sector. For this reason, work requirements and provision of childcare, job training, and other programs to support mothers' transition to employment have come to vary greatly from state to state.[24]

The demand that single mothers take on more paid labor outside the home may seem paradoxical given the prevalent "family values" rhetoric that calls for mothers to forgo or cut back on employment in order to spend more time with their children. However, it is consistent with the gender, class, and race construction of caring labor. The TANF program made explicit what have long been unstated assumptions: that care labor is only properly carried out when it occurs within a self-sufficient male-headed household and that poor women's and women of color's unpaid caring for their families has little social value and does not deserve public support. The fact is that single mothers on welfare have always worked to supplement stingy welfare payments. Thus the expectation and even requirement that single mothers should earn outside income is not a new development.

The earliest public assistance programs for single mothers were Mothers' Pensions, which were established by state legislatures during the Progressive Era. Advocates of Mothers' Pensions such as Edith Abbott, Sophonisba Breckinridge, and Julia Lathrop came from the settlement house movement and were concerned about child welfare and single mothers' economic vulnerability and low wages. They viewed Mothers' Pensions as a means to allow poor women to raise their children at home rather than neglecting them or placing them in orphanages. The Illinois legislature passed the first Mother's Pension law in 1911. Other states soon followed suit, and by 1920, 40 states had such laws.[25]

Contrary to the intents of maternalist advocates, lawmakers and administrators did not intend for Mothers' Pension Programs to allow poor women to stay home with their children. Uniformly stingy in their grants, administrators of Mothers Pensions expected not only mothers but also their children to engage in some form of paid work. For example, in 1913, only two years after its passage, the Mothers' Pension law in Illinois was amended to make work a requirement. The law specified that a mother "may be absent [from home] for work a definite number of days each week to be specified in the court's order." Grants were in fact contingent on recipients working. To determine eligibility, women and their children were examined to determine the extent to which they could work. Linda Gordon notes, "Most mothers' aid recipients, including widows, continued to work for wages, 84 percent in Philadelphia, 66 percent in Chicago and San Francisco, and 57 percent in Los

Angeles." She notes that these figures were underestimated because of the underreporting of women's labor.[26]

Mothers' Pension administrators also applied moral criteria, limiting eligibility only to widows and deserted mothers, so that unmarried (presumably unworthy) mothers were excluded.[27] In making determinations about eligibility, local officials routinely refused pensions to African American and Mexican widows and single mothers. They reasoned that African American mothers were "employable" irrespective of their specific circumstances. They took it for granted that jobs as domestic workers or field hands were always available and that black women should fill these positions as they always had. As for Mexican widows, county officials in Los Angeles argued that the "feudal" background of Mexican immigrants would lead them to "abuse" grants from the state.[28]

A similar pattern characterized the implementation of the Aid to Dependent Children (ADC) program in the 1930s. Depression-era stringencies had all but wiped out state relief programs, including Mother's Pensions. In response to the mounting economic crisis and widespread unemployment, the U.S. Congress passed the Social Security Act (SSA) of 1935 to provide a basic safety net. Social insurance provisions of the SSA included Survivors Insurance for Widows of Workingmen in certain industries. This insurance provided funds sufficient to meet a family's basic needs and did not have any means testing, home inspections, or rules governing the conduct of widows or their children. However, women whose husbands worked in excluded fields such as agriculture and service jobs, as well as women whose husbands had divorced or deserted them, or who were never married, had to rely on public assistance provisions of SSA, in this case Title IV, which created ADC. The program provided one-third of funds allocated by states and counties to implement the program. Title IV attempted to reduce discrimination and broaden coverage by requiring participating states to implement the program in every county and to expand eligibility to include deserted, separated, and unmarried mothers, which only a few state Mothers' Pension programs had allowed.[29]

As in the case of proponents of Mothers' Pensions, early supporters of ADC intended to create a program that would keep single mothers at home to care for their children. Frances Perkins, President Roosevelt's Secretary of Labor, testified to a Senate Committee, "You take the mother of a large family, she may be able-bodied and all that, but we classify her as unemployable because if she works the children have got to go to an orphan asylum."[30] Edith Abbot, Dean of the School of Social Service Administration at the University of Chicago, testified, "These laws are predicated on the theory that long-time care is necessary for these children, that the mother's services are worth more in the home than they are in the outside labor market."[31]

The ADC program was administered by local boards, many of which did not share Perkins's and Abbott's views. A study of ADC in Minneapolis found that the welfare board "made an organized effort to force single girls who are on relief to accept jobs as domestics at home at starvation wages." In several states, including Virginia, South Dakota, and New Jersey, and in Washington, D.C., local welfare offices closed cases when agricultural or domestic jobs were available. In rural areas, able-bodied women were expected to work at harvesting tobacco and cotton, while in urban areas they were directed toward service occupations— as servants, hotel and restaurant workers, cleaners, and laundresses. Yet, administrators of government work programs, such as the Federal Emergency Relief Administration and the Work Projects Administration, deemed single mothers "unemployable," thus closing off these routes to relatively well-paid employment.[32]

African American, Mexican American, and other mothers of color were more likely to be denied eligibility than white women. In 1943, Louisiana implemented an "employable mother" rule that any capable woman with a child over 7 years of age should be denied assistance if there was fieldwork available. Georgia adopted a similar rule in 1951 that required able-bodied women with children over the age of 3 to work when "suitable work" was available. In both cases, the rules were intended to disqualify black women. By 1962, 33 states had inserted work requirements in their ADC regulations; many of these states cut off aid to any recipient who refused a job offer.[33]

After World War II, the rise of black civil rights activism, mass migration of African Americans to northern cities, and the increase in African Americans on urban welfare rolls (even though the majority of welfare recipients were white) gave rise to increasing attacks on welfare. In 1960 the Louisiana legislature passed a "suitable home" law that instantly disqualified 23,000 predominately black children born out of wedlock from receiving ADC. The law was part of a biannual packet of "segregation" bills designed to keep blacks "in their place." The Louisiana actions garnered national attention only when, alerted by U.S. activists, an English city council in Newcastle-on-Tyne organized an airlift of baby food to feed the children of New Orleans. A year later, the city manager of Newburgh, New York, Joseph Mitchell, enacted harsh cutbacks on welfare, limiting assistance to 3 months and setting stringent work requirements. Newburgh's actions attracted national attention and widespread support.[34]

According to Lisa Levenstein, these events turned welfare into a smoldering public issue, placing it at the center of racial politics and making "public assistance into a scapegoat for the nation's ills for the first time, but not the last."[35] Even among supporters of ADC, public assistance came to be seen less as a means to ensure that poor single mothers could care for their own children and more as a means by which black women could avoid employment. President John F. Kennedy proposed and Congress passed a series of amendments to SSA that mandated that the program, renamed Aid to Families of Dependent Children (AFDC), expend more for job training and counseling for welfare clients and provide "work incentives" for women on assistance.[36]

These work incentives became required for states with the passage of the 1967 amendments to the Social Security Act, which created the Work Incentive Program (WIN) that encouraged employment by providing education, job training, and structured job searches that recipients carried out and reported back on efforts to find work. Importantly, it allowed recipients of AFDC to keep part of their earnings. Even at peak funding in 1980 ($350 million), WIN provided only $250 to serve each potential recipient. Susan Blank and Barbara Blum note that "Operating the WIN employment and training programs cost welfare agencies more than issuing monthly benefit checks, so WIN became little more than a registration requirement for many recipients."[37]

With the rise of the civil rights movement in the 1960s, welfare recipients and their advocates became active players, organizing under the banner of "welfare rights." Their efforts, as revealed in their self-designation, were aimed at asserting economic support for poor women and children as an entitlement and ending racial discrimination in welfare policy and enforcement. Civil rights and anti-poverty lawyers filed suit in courts challenging state regulations that disqualified many poor women and had discriminatory work requirements. These suits resulted in a few victories, notably overturning regulations that denied assistance to full-time workers. However, the courts upheld the right of individual states to set work requirements, including requirements that were more stringent than those mandated by the federal government. Strict work requirements functioned to deny coverage to many poor women, thus impeding their opportunity to care for their own children full-time.[38]

Another effort to reshape welfare policy occurred in 1988, with the passage of the Family Support Act (FSA) of 1988. The FSA created a new state-operated program known as Job Opportunities and Basic Skills (JOBS), which was designed to move more AFDC recipients from welfare to work by matching state contributions for child care, by increasing child care subsidies, and by continuing child care and Medicaid subsidies for a year after the transition to paid employment. However, funding for the JOBS program depended on individual states' willingness to put up their own funds in order to receive a federal match. Most states failed to claim all of the federal dollars to which they were entitled. In 1993, nearly one-third of the $1 billion of available federal funds went unclaimed. The success of JOBS programs varied hugely, depending on local leadership and initiative. The General Accounting Office reported that in 1992 only one-fourth of eligible recipients were engaged in JOBS activities in any given month.[39]

How does the history of governmental efforts to get women off welfare and into work outside the home relate to poor women's unpaid caring under the 1996 Temporary Aid to Needy Families (TANF) program? Many critics of TANF have charged that it represented a radical shift from an earlier time when mothers caring for minor children were held in high regard and deemed worthy of public support. As the foregoing history shows, respect for mothers caring at home was never unalloyed. Public assistance programs consistently treated African American mothers' caring as less worthy than that of white mothers. Moreover, the ideal of full-time motherhood has coexisted with the doctrine of family self-sufficiency. The two are congruent within the context of a male-headed household in which economic support and caring are divided along gender lines. They conflict when mothers and children lack a male breadwinner, and mothers are then expected to take on earning as well as caring in order to make the family self-supporting. Advocates of Mothers' Pensions and ADC understood that low-wage employment posed a serious obstacle to mothers being able to support their children and that therefore the economic value of mothers' care work in the home was greater than the earnings their labor could command in the market. But, as we have seen, once enacted, the programs focused not on making it possible for single mothers to care for their children but instead on compelling them to fulfill their parental obligation to earn.

The stated goals of the 1996 Personal Responsibility and Work Opportunity Reconciliation Act (PRWORA), which created the TANF program, were to reduce dependence of low-income families on government aid, promote employment and self-sufficiency, promote marriage, and reduce births outside of marriage. The TANF program differed from previous AFDC welfare-to-work programs by placing time limits on assistance—five years over a lifetime—and requiring recipients to make efforts toward paid employment within two years. PRWORA established benchmark "work participation rates" for states, starting at 25 percent and rising to 50 percent by 2002, and provided incentives to states to reduce welfare rolls in the form of "caseload reduction credits." These credits could be used to offset work participation rates, thus creating an incentive for states to remove recipients from the rolls and deny new applicants.[40]

The most visible short-term "success" of the TANF program was to reduce welfare rolls. Surveys and studies of case loads in the four-year period after the TANF program was created found that the number of recipients fell by 6.5 million, more than a 53 percent drop, with a further 300,000 fewer recipients in the fifth year. This five-year period was one of economic expansion, so there is some question about how much of the decline was caused by welfare reform. Indeed, caseloads had fallen by 18 percent in the three-year period leading up to the passage of PRWORA, partly because of state-level reforms but mostly because of favorable economic conditions.[41]

Of course, measuring the success of welfare reform solely by reduction in welfare rolls is similar to measuring success of deinstitutionalization solely by the fact that there are fewer people in institutions without taking into account the increase in homelessness. In neither case does it mean that those who are no longer included are doing better; it only means they're not being counted. Using data from the 2002

National Survey of American Families, Gregory Acs and Pamela Loprest estimated that 19 percent of recipients who left the welfare rolls could be described as "disconnected." That is, they were not on TANF, not employed, not living with a working spouse or partner, and not on disability. Who are these "dropouts"? Acs and Loprest confirmed that most are women who confront multiple barriers to employment. More than 30 percent have poor physical or mental health, 38 percent have less than a high school education, 47 percent have last worked more than three years previously; 8 percent have a child under 1; and 20 percent have a child with a disability who receives Supplemental Security Income.[42]

In the absence of public assistance and steady earnings, poor women have historically turned to informal sources of assistance such as occasional gifts from a child's father, loans of cash from a sister, or emergency housing from an uncle. These "informal" sources of assistance are as irregular and impermanent as welfare or the kinds of jobs that are most readily available; they can disappear suddenly if a partner gets arrested, a sister loses her job, or an uncle loses his apartment. Receiving assistance from family also entails reciprocal obligations, so it usually involves adding to the amount of unpaid labor that single mothers must perform.

As to transition from welfare to employment, studies conducted in the first few years after the TANF program was created found a substantial rate of employment (60 percent) for those who left welfare and a rise in employment (28 percent) among those still receiving aid.[43] The vast majority of employment was low-wage, slightly above minimum wage; even though averaging 35 hours a week, overall wages averaged about two-thirds of the federal poverty line for families. Three-quarters of workers received no vacation or sick days, and more than half were without medical benefits.[44] Over a quarter worked mostly night hours, during which it is difficult to find child care coverage.[45] Studies of the jobs held by recipients and former recipients in Maryland, South Carolina, Washington State, and Wisconsin found that a majority of former recipients worked in food preparation, sales, clerical support, or other service sector jobs.[46] As Sharon Hayes summarizes the situation, "The problem for most welfare clients, then, is not getting a job, but finding a job that pays enough to bring the family out of poverty, offers benefits, and is flexible enough to make room for the circumstances of single parenting. The odds of finding that job—and keeping it—are not good when you are a woman with low skills and children to care for."[47]

Several major large-scale studies collected data on urban and rural poor families over several years following the implementation of the TANF program. These studies yielded rich quantitative information and ethnographic observations that bear on such important questions as whether welfare recipients have been able to remain employed for sustained periods of time; whether families are financially better off when mothers are employed instead of on welfare; and how mothers' employment affects children's well-being. Additionally, these data have been used to assess the effectiveness of specific provisions within the TANF program to encourage marriage and discourage births outside of marriage.[48]

Of central concern for this volume are two questions: How have work requirements and time limits affected the amount, form, and quality of care that single mothers provide for their children? And, to what extent do single mothers feel they are able to provide the kind of care they want for their children? Interviews with poor single mothers reveal that they subscribe to the widely held ideal of self-sufficiency. Moreover, women on welfare agree with advocates of reform that single mothers should work to support themselves and their children and that they ought not to expect others who are employed to support them.[49] It is thus not surprising that mothers who have transitioned to jobs report that they have greater self-esteem than when they were not employed. Mothers' attitudes are echoed by adolescent children, who, perhaps aware of the stigma attached to being on welfare, report feeling better about themselves when mothers are employed.[50]

Single mothers simultaneously subscribe to the dominant ideal of motherhood, which stresses the importance of mothers being attentive and available, especially in the early years of a child's life. Laura Lein and her co-authors observe:

> At the core of mothers' experiences with the labor force lies a conflict. Almost universally, mothers make mothering their top priority. While policy makers might argue that self-sufficiency is a primary value, for the mothers we talked to, being a good parent comes first. Mothers weighed the possibilities provided in the labor force against the needs of their children. The greatest needs for which they contended were

for a stable and consistent home and, perhaps even more, a way of life that was secure, providing the necessities of daily living in a regular and predictable fashion.[51]

Poor mothers' prioritizing mothering over employment needs to be understood in the context of their experiences in the labor market. They value "self-sufficiency" but often do not see their low-wage jobs making them self-sufficient.[52] The kinds of jobs they typically can get are low-waged, often part-time and/or temporary, and offer no vacation time or health insurance. More than half of all mothers transitioning to work enter the service sector, which is characterized by irregular hours and lack of benefits. These kinds of jobs do not offer sick days or flexibility to allow for such contingencies as a child getting sick or problems with child care. In such cases, mothers give priority to their child's interests; they may not show up for work and so get fired, or they may decide it is not worth jeopardizing their children's well-being and quit. Andrew London and his colleagues report on the case of Toni, a 20-year-old white mother of two, who explained why she gave up her job at a suburban McDonald's:

At first I started off in the morning time. . . . I had somebody watching my children and they wasn't picking my son up on time from school. . . . He was going to get put out of the program. So I switched to nighttime so that I could pick him up. And then I was making him late to school because I was so tired. I was getting in the house like 1:30–2:00 . . . and I couldn't get up in the morning to get him ready for school. So, I just tried to get back to daytime and they didn't have room and that was it.[53]

Because they place a high priority on their children's needs, having high-quality child care while working is an important and difficult issue. The TANF program supposedly includes subsidies for child care during the first year of employment. However, some experts have found that most mothers eligible for subsidies do not receive them,[54] so single mothers have to patch together child care. Because of the length of their work days and long commutes, nearly two-thirds of full-time low-income working mothers in Chicago "relied heavily on at least two caregivers (in addition to themselves) during the course of their children's typical day." Single mothers who had kin who were willing and able to provide child care assistance (e.g., watching after children before or after school, giving them snacks and meals, accompanying them from school to an after-school program) were most able not only to get jobs but to keep them. Roy, Tubbs, and Burton note, "Almost every mother arranged for almost all of her children to spend part of the day with a family member." Mothers reported that their own mothers provided the bulk of child care assistance.[55] Although it is undoubtedly true that grandmothers enjoy spending time with their grandchildren, in this case their childcare labor is "obligatory"—a status duty. If they do not provide assistance, their daughters will not be able to work, and their grandchildren will suffer. By performing unpaid child care, they are subsidizing the low-wage system and relieving the state and the employer from having to pay for the cost of social reproduction.

Many single mothers who have taken outside jobs complain that they do not get to spend enough time with their children. These women have the same ideals as other mothers, that parents should see their children off to school, spend mealtimes with them, oversee their homework, and read them bedtime stories. Even those who say that they have gained financially or psychologically from employment fear that their relationships with their children suffer because they have less time to spend with them. Celeste, a single mother interviewed for a 2004 study by Andrew London and colleagues, recognized the benefits of working, saying "The income is much better, and they [my four children] can get more and they're more proud of me and I'm proud of myself." However, she also spoke of loss—the loss of time with her children: "You know sometimes when they come home, cause I have to be at work by 5, so I leave at 4. When they come home from school I'm right out the door. I just give them a kiss, and I don't have that time with them no more." Danielle, a mother of two stated that the costs of work for her children outweighed the benefits: "I feel better when I go to work. . . . I like being around people. I just wish I didn't have to work so long. . . . I think I should be home when my kids get out of school, I should be here with them. But I'm not, who knows where my kids will grow up and go . . . what way they're gonna turn."[56]

That these mothers' experiences are common is confirmed by the 2003 study by Chase-Landale et al. of 2,402 low-income children and mothers in Boston, Chicago, and San Antonio. According to time-use diaries kept by mothers, preschoolers "experienced a significant decline in time spent with their mothers. When mothers moved into employment, they decreased total time with their preschoolers by an average of 2.1 hours a day." As for adolescent children, Chase-Landale et al. noted: "There is some evidence in the literature showing that mothers are able to compensate for time away from [adolescent] children due to employment by cutting down on sleep, leisure or volunteer activities, and our time-use data suggest that when mothers went to work, they cut back on personal, social and educational activities that did not involve their children."[57] This giving up of "personal projects" and time for oneself is similar to the sacrifices made by family caregivers of medical technology–dependent children and spouses and helps explain the high levels of stress, tiredness, and anxiety that poor working women report.

Tubbs, Burton, and Roy's 2005 investigation of time use in low-income African American, Latina, and white families in Chicago further fills out the picture by showing the ways mothers juggle multiple demands and carve out "family time" with their children. The mothers made special efforts to engage their children in talk, spend mealtimes with them, provide treats, and play with them in the course of daily activities. The authors noted, for example, "Working single mothers in particular intentionally sat down to family meals with their children but did not eat with them. Their work schedules were not synchronized to their children's mealtimes, so although they were home during their children's dinner, their typical dinner meal occurred prior to or after the children's dinner time." Barbara, a 35-year-old single parent with two young children reported that she mostly snacked during the day rather than sitting down to meals. She added, "even in the evening when I do eat, I probably wait (until) after the kids have eaten. I want to make sure they've eaten." Another single mother, Cherry, said "I don't eat, I am telling you; I can't because I need to make sure this one does his homework . . . and this one doesn't go outside and cut out on me, and I need to makes sure (this one) is okay. I might get a bit here or there, but I don't really eat."[58]

Another analysis by the same researchers showed that working single mothers sacrificed employment opportunities and their own health to maintain their children's well-being. Yolanda, the mother of a kindergartner and a sixth grader, worked in a paper factory while her children were in school. Her children went to different after-school programs, an arrangement that was difficult in terms of transportation and problematic for the children, who wanted to be together in day care. To pay for better after-school day care that both could attend, Yolanda took a third shift job delivering papers from 1:00 a.m. to 5:00 a.m. while her children slept. Low-income mothers often had long commutes on public transportation, prolonging time away from children. Barbara stayed at home and cared for her children during the day. "After preparing and serving dinner, she caught public transportation to the suburbs where she worked in a large package-loading company. Unfortunately, the suburban bus system and Chicago's bus and train system are not synchronized, with suburban buses unavailable when she finished her shift. She waited 2–3 hours for the first morning bus 3 days each week." Barbara confessed, "I always fall asleep on the (Chicago city) bus—I gotta stop that. Miss my stop."[59]

As these examples indicate, sleeping is one of the things single working mothers sacrificed to accommodate employment and caring. Tubbs and her colleagues found that 20 percent of low-income mothers had "non-normative sleep patterns," catching some sleep during the day; many had "split schedules" in which their sleep was briefly interrupted by childcare or household duties. Tubbs et al. note that most mothers sacrificed personal time by giving a high priority to time with their children. "'My time' typically occurred late at night after the children were asleep or during a nap, often in front of the TV." The authors conclude that employment requirements have forced poor women to integrate multiple time demands into their schedules. "In a sense, as their temporal orientations have shifted, low income mothers have lost control over how to allocate family time, and at times even endanger their own health through inadequate diet, sleep deprivation, and elevated depression and anxiety."[60]

All of these findings speak to the fragility of poor single women's "self sufficiency through employment" and the contingent nature of their ability to care for their children while employed. Low-income mothers are better able to sustain employment if they are physically and mentally healthy and their children do not have chronic conditions or behavioral problems *and* they have considerable informal support from family and kin, because they receive little or nothing in the way of public assistance. Mothers with multiple problems and inadequate informal support experience greater overload and negative spillover between family care and work. Under these conditions, which are all too common, they cannot sustain employment over the long run.[61] For poor women the issue is not the one that welfare reform has promised—that parents' employment is a precondition for family well-being; rather the issue is that a fundamental level of family well-being—including time and energy for caring—is a precondition for successful parental employment.[62]

Commodifying Care

Even as the amount of time and effort that women have been forced to devote to unpaid home health care for family members has increased, and as poor women's energies are being diverted from caring labor in the home to paid employment, there has also been greater reliance on the services of paid home-care workers.

As we have seen, federal and state policies favor non-institutional care for the elderly and disabled and also assume that family members will provide a great deal of unpaid care. However, policy makers increasingly recognize that paid home care is often needed to supplement informal care in order to keep disabled children and adults and frail elderly out of institutions. Many states have developed programs to provide home care for low-income children, parents, seniors, and people with disabilities either through direct payments to clients or through public or private home-care organizations.

The biggest source of public funds for home health and personal care comes from the joint federal–state Medicaid program, which instituted Home Health Services as a mandatory benefit for individuals who are entitled to care in a nursing home and added Personal Care Services (PCS) as an optional benefit in 1993. As of 2005, 26 states and the District of Columbia offered the PCS benefit.[63] Medicaid legislation also contains a waiver program that allows states to provide services not usually covered by Medicaid "as long as these services are required to keep a person from being institutionalized."[64] Every state offers home-care services, with most operating under these waiver provisions. States may set their own eligibility criteria but must conform to federal guidelines in order to receive grants and matching funds. As a consequence of Home Health Services, the Home Care Benefit waiver, and Personal Care Service benefits, the allocation of Medicaid funding for long-term care shifted substantially from institutional to home care. According to an AARP analysis, by 2005, more than one-third (37 percent) of Medicaid funding for long-term care was spent on home care. Out of total

Medicare spending on long-term care of $94.5 billion in 2005, $59.5 billion was spent on institutional care, and $35.0 billion was spent on home care.[65]

The growing demand for home care and the increased availability of state funds during the period before the recession that began in 2008 fueled growth in the market for paid home care. This growth was reflected in the rising numbers of those employed in providing direct care and in the proliferation of third-party entities that broker home-care services. However, in at least some states (such as California) this growth may be endangered by drastic cuts in state-funded home-care programs for 2010 and future years.

The U.S. Department of Labor (DOL) divides paid home-care workers into two categories, home health aides (who provide personal care with bathing, toileting, and dressing) and personal and home-care aides (who provide assistance with daily living activities such as housekeeping and preparing meals). According to a recent DOL report, 1.55 million workers were employed in these two occupations in 2007.[66] This number was expected to mushroom for reasons discussed above. DOL experts have projected the two occupations to be among the fastest-growing jobs in the United States, with an increase of 48.7 percent in home health aides and 50.6 percent in personal and home-care aides between 2006 and 2016, at which time 2.33 million workers are expected to be employed in these occupations.[67] All of these counts almost certainly underestimate the actual numbers of home-care workers, since, as will be noted below, a goodly portion of the home-care labor market is underground—part of the so-called "gray market."

A second effect of the boom in paid home care has been the proliferation of home-care brokers. Some of this demand is being met by non-profit organizations, such as visiting nurse associations, which have set up special divisions to provide home care to paying clients, and by public agencies such as those that administer California's In Home Support Services program at the county level.[68] Another type of non-profit is the worker cooperative, the model for which is the Cooperative Home Care Associates (CHCA), located in South Bronx, New York. CHCA was founded in 1985 with the dual purpose of providing quality home care and providing quality jobs for women wanting to leave welfare. It has contracts with state agencies to provide home-care services and currently provides jobs for 1,600 individuals.[69]

The most striking development, one that is typical of the neoliberal privatization of welfare, has been the entry of profit-making corporations into the field of home care. Their entry has been made possible by policies whereby state agencies administering programs for disabled and elderly contract services to outside entities, including profit-making companies. These companies recruit, screen, train, and employ workers who are sent out to care in recipient's homes. The availability of private health insurance dollars and federal Medicaid funds with which states and counties can pay for home health care and personal care at home has created a stream of income upon which corporations can draw.

The for-profit sector of home care, in turn, is stratified to serve different socioeconomic segments of the market. At the high end are full-service agencies that offer supervised home health and personal care for affluent seniors who can afford premium service or whose care expenses are covered by corporate employee assistance programs or long-term care insurance. Two examples are the SeniorBridge company that operates in 15 locations in the Northeast, as well as in Chicago, San Antonio, and Florida, and HouseWorks, a Boston firm that has been identified by the *New York Times* as "a boutique agency with fewer than 700 clients and gross revenues of $9 million." These upscale companies offer trained and supervised home care aides as one part of an array of home medical and health services provided by nurses, social workers, nutrition and exercise specialists, and home health and care aides, all overseen by a care manager.[70]

Competing for clients of more modest means are local home-care companies that offer only non-medical services. They cater to recently discharged patients and seniors requiring ongoing assistance, offering such services as light laundry and housekeeping, meal preparation, and escorting to doctor's appointments. Clients pay out of pocket or from Medicaid allowances. Many private firms are part of chain franchises. In exchange for franchise fees, the franchiser provides training in running home-care businesses, for example, how to recruit home-care workers and how to market and attract clients. One of the largest franchisers is Home Instead, which claims to have more than 700 "independently owned and operated franchisers [sic]" and to employ 37,000 part-time care workers tending to 43,000 elderly clients. Visiting Angels, founded in 1998, claims 300 home franchisees in 46 states.[71]

Even with these increased options, according to a *New York Times* article in 2007, more and more families are turning to the underground "gray market" to find affordable care. One might well intuit that the simultaneous entry of corporate investors and entrepreneurs into the home-care market and the development of a substantial underground economy around home care are interrelated consequences of present-day neoliberal economic policy.[72] In global cities such as New York, we find both a booming corporation-dominated formal economy alongside a vibrant underground economy, and growing affluence alongside rising poverty. Poor families and individuals have often had to work in or acquire goods and services from the underground economy to get by. What seems new is that many affluent middle-class families that do not ordinarily participate in the underground economy are doing so when they look for household help and for home care for their parents.

Clients use the gray market to avoid having to pay agency fees. For example, in New York State, a bonded, insured, and certified agency worker cost $24 an hour (of which $8.22 went to the worker), while a gray-market caregiver could be hired for half the agency rate.[73] For clients, the advantage of using the gray market is that they can afford more hours of care; for care workers, the advantage is that they can often earn more per hour and avoid deductions for taxes, although it sometimes means giving up Social Security and health insurance. Clients and care workers link up through informal referrals among friends and neighbors.[74] The main drawback for clients is the lack of formal screening, background checks, or training; however, they may also feel more comfortable when a caregiver has been "vouched for" by someone in their personal network rather than when a "stranger" has been sent by an impersonal company. Moreover, experienced home-care workers are often part of immigrant communities and/or have worked in agencies and nursing homes and know other caregivers. They can thus offer stability and flexible coverage by being able to recruit a relative or a friend to replace them, substitute during vacation time, or provide additional hours if the elder gets sick and needs more hours of care.[75]

I offer my own experience as an example of the workings of the gray market. In 2005 I was seeking home care for my mother, who needed assistance while recuperating from a back injury after falling on a bus. She needed assistance with showering, meal preparation, light housework, and laundry. During a few initial inquiries to organizations in the local Japanese American community, I was advised that the most common and effective way to find a caregiver was to ask around my friends and acquaintances. An acquaintance who ran a twice-monthly senior program at a local church gave me the name of a Filipina woman, Julita,[76] who had taken care of a senior from her program. Julita was an experienced caregiver, middle aged with a sunny personality and a take-charge attitude. She was listed with a local hospital as a home health aide for recently discharged patients and also did freelance home care. My friend had told me that I would have to pay $16 to $18 an hour, and Julita said she would charge $16 if it was "under the table." I decided I would prefer to employ her legally and pay for social security and unemployment insurance, but once Julita met my mother, she agreed to work "on the books" for $16 anyway. For the first two months, we wanted to have someone with my mother around the clock "just in case." Julita said she could sleep in at night because she had a day job already and offered to find other women to work during the day hours. She introduced us to Malea, a young Filipina, and to Haben, an Eritrean immigrant woman, both of whom she knew through the local hospital. Julita asked us to make out any checks owed to Malea to her, and she would pay Malea. Haben had a sister, Naeema, who had recently arrived from Eritrea and needed a job; she was only beginning to learn English, but after a couple of weeks, Naeema took Haben's place. Later, when my mother needed only a few hours a day of help, Malea and Naeema took alternate days. Eventually Malea got a job as a cashier at a drugstore, and Naeema worked four hours a day, six days a week to help with meals, to accompany my mother on walks, and to take her shopping. Julita in the meantime started working full-time caring for the mother of the woman who had originally recommended her to me.

As the case of these caregivers indicates, formal and gray markets for home care are not completely separate. Some care workers, like Julita and Haben combine part-time private sector work and gray market work to get enough hours to support themselves. Other workers, such as Malea, who would not qualify for agency work and are not certified, work only in the gray market. These workers are not included in official statistics on home-care aides and home health aides, so their numbers cannot be ascertained. However, anecdotal evidence suggests that they are very numerous and that they are heavily made up of immigrant women, with the largest representations from Latin America, the Philippines, Africa, and the Caribbean.

Although clients, public agencies, and for-profit firms lament the shortage of home-care workers, they have not raised wages and benefits to attract more workers. To the contrary, Medicaid and other programs limit hourly wage rates, often to federal or state minimum wage levels. Home health aides and home-care aides remain among the lowest paid of all occupations, with average wages for home health aides of $9.66 an hour and for home care aides of $8.74. These earnings are about half of the average for all workers of $18.84. With full-time, year-round work, home health aides would earn an average of $20,100, while home-care aides would earn $18,180, both with virtually no benefits. However, even these figures are misleading because two-thirds of home care workers do not work full-time the year around.[77] This is in part because Medicaid and insurance programs restrict the number of hours they will cover for each care receiver. Consequently, workers typically care for two or more clients each day to piece together an income. They are not paid for time spent traveling from one home to another, which can be considerable. Not surprisingly, the average home care worker's earnings was about two-thirds of full time, so that the average earnings of many were well below the official poverty line. A U.S. General Accounting Office report found that nearly one in five (18.8 percent) care workers had incomes that were below the poverty line, and more than one in seven (14.8 percent) received food stamps.[78]

Who Are the Paid Home-Care Workers?

The consequence of low wages and challenging work conditions is that few women or men choose home-care work if they have other options. As a result, the ranks of home-care workers are disproportionately made up of those whose choices are limited. One picture can be gleaned from official sources. U.S. Census data indicate that paid personal and home-care aides are overwhelmingly women (91.8 percent). They are disproportionately immigrants (24.9 percent), and whether immigrant or native, half are people of color (49.7 percent). Home-care workers are also likely to be older (median age of 46) and to have lower levels of education (30.9 percent with less than high school) than workers in other occupations.[79]

Because workers in the gray market are not accounted for in U.S. Census data, their composition may differ from those who are in the formal economy. It seems likely that newly arrived immigrants, especially undocumented immigrants, form a much higher percentage of those in the home-care gray market than those who are included in the Census. Domestic service including home care in the gray market is one of the few readily available jobs for undocumented women because they do not have the papers necessary to sign up with an agency or home-care company. As a Filipina undocumented immigrant in New York City working unofficially explained:

> My options were limited, my priorities were very clear: support my children, give them a better future, and then to support myself. My only realistic option was to work, and work meant anything that the system will allow. If you don't have work authorization you can't find things—even if you have education and skill. So that's how Philippines [sic] become domestic workers here. It's not a choice. It's not the best option for us but you do it to survive and support our families.[80]

Employers may prefer immigrant women not only because they are cheaper but also because they view them as superior caregivers. They view women from the global south as coming from traditional cultures in which families honor and take care of the elderly. Employers feel that they are more likely to work without complaining and show proper deference. Further, the immigrant's lack of citizenship makes her more "pliable" and controllable. Thus, employers can more easily take advantage of the worker. Immigrant care workers often face the problem of "job creep," being expected to take on additional tasks beyond those originally agreed upon. One care worker recalled, "You have to deal with the family, who maybe wants you to do their work, like the laundry and going shopping, and that's not what you're there for. If they don't clean up you have to clean up but you're only supposed to be cleaning the area around the patient. You get accused of things you didn't do."[81]

As in early twentieth-century relations between housewives and servants, the employment of immigrant women in home care often involves a division of labor in which the main task of family members is to organize and monitor paid caregivers who perform the physical, hands-on "dirty" work. More affluent women fulfill their obligation to care by delegating the more onerous and time-consuming aspects of their caring obligation. And, as in the case of domestic service, paid home-care labor actually reinforces the gender division of caring labor; it also helps maintain the myth of the private family as the realm of caring and dependency and justifies the family-centered care model in which wives/daughters/ mothers are ultimately responsible for the care of family members. Employing women from "traditional" cultures is particularly effective in "familizing" paid care work. If caring is viewed as a cultural trait or a natural attribute of women from Latin America, Africa, and Asia, then their labor can be seen as effortless and not real work. Thus, even though they are working for pay, immigrant caregivers help to sustain the ideal of informal family care.[82]

We can see that all of the larger trends in the global economy converge in shaping the situation of paid home-care workers: In the global north these forces include the outsourcing of production; the increasing reliance on the service sector for economic growth; the feminization of paid labor; low reproduction rates with consequent aging of the population; neoliberal economic policy such as downsizing the welfare state; and increasing income inequality. In the global south, these forces include economic "reforms" imposed by international financial institutions that have led to reduction of state welfare, selling off of state-run enterprises, and destruction of subsistence agriculture in favor of monoculture of export crops.[83]

Having lost their traditional means of livelihood and even minimal government safety nets, large segments of the rural populations in the global south have turned to transnational migration in search of work so as to support their families. A substantial portion of female migrants to the global north have found work in the service sector, including cleaning, domestic service, and home care. Like other migrant workers, they send remittances to their families in their home countries, thereby helping to keep their families and their countries afloat. For some ailing economies, such as those of the Philippines, Mexico, El Salvador, Guatemala, Algeria, Turkey, and Albania, remittances from migrants working abroad constitute a substantial portion of national incomes. In the countries where they migrate, their labor helps to bridge the contradiction between social policy that places responsibility for the care of citizens on families rather than the state and economic policies that have reduced the capacity of families to provide unpaid care, for example, by forcing members, including mothers, to devote more time to paid employment. In short, migrant care workers are central to the maintenance of families and economies in both north and south.[84]

The social organization of caring labor has emerged as a vastly complex and variegated structure that spans the boundaries of the "private" and the "public" spheres and brings the market directly and powerfully into the home. This structure also crosses national boundaries, transferring care labor from the global south to homes in the global north. Whereas in the past, caring was largely taken for granted as belonging in the private family sphere and as an activity natural to women, we see that the way in which it is organized and carried out is far from "natural" but rather is shaped by political and economic forces, social policy, and popular discourse. We can nonetheless see significant indications of continuity in the imposition of coercion, even if the outward appearance of the forms may have changed. Today, more women than ever before are being forced to care, in new and problematic ways.

7

Creating a Caring Society

The most visible facet of the care crisis in the United States and other developed societies is the so-called care deficit. The number of those needing care—the elderly, disabled, and other dependents—has risen sharply in recent decades while the ranks of those who have tradition-ally provided care have thinned. As a result, many of our most vul-nerable citizens are not receiving the amount or quality of care they need and deserve. Family members and friends are overburdened with caring responsibilities and are too often sacrificing their own health and well-being to provide care for their loved ones. Paid caregivers, many of whom are recent immigrants and minority women of color, toil for low wages, without protections and benefits, and with little prospect of security and dignity in their old age. These two situations are in sub-stantial danger of becoming even more perilous with draconian cuts in government-provided funding for home-care services, as mandated by states such as California for its 2010 and future budgets.

My focus in this book is to understand long-standing structural and ideological underpinnings of the crisis affecting those needing care, those providing unpaid care, and those providing paid care. I have re-ferred to these structural and ideological underpinnings under the general rubric of the social organization of care. Three general features have characterized caring in our society. First, caring has been orga-nized around spatial and conceptual separation between public and private realms. The public sphere of the market (economy and politics) and the private sphere of family and household are imagined to be dis-crete arenas that serve different purposes, perform different functions, and operate according to different principles. Success in the public sphere is thought to require people to be independent so that they can engage in competition and pursue self-interest; this conception requires the exclusion of dependency needs from the public sphere and their sequestration within the so-called private sphere. The family is thus viewed as the proper location for meeting dependency needs, and family members are charged with responsibility for taking care of one another. This principle is embedded in everyday mores and internalized as a status obligation, such that individuals feel morally obligated on the basis of a parental, child, or spousal relationship. It is also incorporated into law and social policy, which, for example, has denied the right to compensation for caring for family members and withheld state subsidized care for those who have close kin nearby. Because kin are assumed to be fulfilling strictly personal responsibility, kin care labor is not considered real work, and the lack of monetary compensation for it means that kin care does not fulfill one's citizenship duty to earn and support oneself. Thus, to the extent that individuals reduce paid employment in order to take on more unpaid caring for relatives, they forgo benefits and recognition that are tied to working and earning.

A second structural feature of caring labor is that gender, class, race, and citizenship status are central axes in the social organization of caring. Concretely, this means that the burden of care (including both the responsibility for it and the actual labor) is differentially distributed according to gender, class, race, and citizenship. The pattern of women taking disproportionate responsibility for care is so well established that it is largely taken for granted, often not noticed, and, when noticed, seen as natural. Also taken for granted is the pattern of poor people, people of color, and immigrants providing care for more affluent native-born whites. Further, as with other types of labor, caring is subject to division into higher and lower levels: more spiritual versus more menial tasks, more intellectual versus more physical duties, and more supervisory versus more hands-on work. Poor people, people of color, and noncitizens are charged with a greater share of the menial, physical, and hands-on work of care. Thus the low status of caring work and the low status of care workers are mutually reinforced.

The third structural feature is that care and non-care labor have different relationships to freedom and coercion. Recruitment into caring has historically relied on coercion, either direct or indirect. Historically, caring has been associated with lack of freedom, with caring labor drawn from those restricted by slavery, indenture, colonialism, caste, social and spatial segregation, and other systems of exclusion and containment. We do not deny the intrinsic rewards of caring, but the features of separation of public and private spheres and the inequalities related to gender, class, and race have meant there was little material incentive to do this work. Moreover, demand does not increase the price of care labor. In this sense, paid caring labor is expected to operate outside of the vaunted market principles valorized by economists. In the absence of significant material benefits, there is little to attract people into care work; instead, restrictions that cut off other options and "tracking" mechanisms seem to be the primary impetuses for entry into care work.

In all three areas, social structure and ideology reinforce one another. For example, economic restructuring has displaced men and women from subsistence activities in the global south, impelling them to migrate to the global north in search of work; once in the north, legal, educational, and labor market barriers severely limit immigrants' occupational options. Simultaneously, the dominant ideology portrays immigrant women of color as "naturally" subservient because of gender, race, and culture. Historically, social and legal restrictions on middle-class married women kept them out of the public realm of politics and the professions and constrained them to the private sphere of the family, while ideologies of home, motherhood, and respectable womanhood exalted their role as caregivers. As discussed earlier, during the nineteenth and early twentieth centuries, American territorial expansion and subjugation of Native Americans and colonial subjects were premised on an ideology that posed a dichotomy between civilized and uncivilized peoples. A cornerstone of so-called civilized societies was the "Christian family," with its clearly differentiated masculine and feminine roles, with men acting as household heads and economic providers and women dedicating themselves to domesticity, including care for children and the elderly. Part of the aim of civilizing subject peoples was to reform their domestic practices by inducting their women into domestic service. Remnants of these older ideologies of servitude and entitlement tied to social status cling to caring relationships today.

These prevalent patterns in social structure and ideology are pervasive and deep-seated and are not easily reformed.

Toward a Caring Society

This book is not intended to generate specific policy recommendations. Rather, by excavating the ideological and structural bases for the current care crisis and the dilemmas faced by unpaid family carers, we can begin to rethink fundamental assumptions and taken-for-granted practices about care. Because the social organization of care work is grounded in the inherited inequalities of the U.S. economic and legal systems, as well as those in the contemporary global system, and given the deeply held and unexamined personal and social attitudes about caring, it is a challenge to imagine major changes in the way caring work is treated in the United States.

In order to develop alternatives to the present inequitable (and ultimately unworkable) situation, we need to rethink the concept of care. Because care is so closely associated with womanhood, feminist philosophers and social theorists have subjected care to close analysis. Theorists of care, including Joan Tronto, Dietmut Bubeck, Emily Abel and Margaret Nelson, and Sara Ruddick, suggest the usefulness of thinking of care as a practice that encompasses feeling (caring about) and activity (caring for). "Caring about" engages both thought and emotion, including awareness and attentiveness, concern about and feelings of responsibility for meeting another's needs. "Caring for" refers to the varied activities of providing for the needs or well-being of another person.[1] These activities include physical care (e.g., bathing, feeding), emotional care (e.g., reassuring, sympathetic listening), and direct services (e.g., driving a person to the doctor, running errands). These definitions are not free of ambiguity, but they do establish some boundaries. For example, defining caring in terms of direct meeting of needs differentiates caring from other activities that may foster survival. Thus economic provision would not be included, even though it may help to support caregiving. Men are often said to be "taking care of their family" when they earn and bring money into the household. Despite the use of the word "care" in this phrase, breadwinning would not be considered as "caring"; in fact, economic support has historically been seen as men's contribution in lieu of actual caregiving. Simultaneously, caregiving has been viewed as women's responsibility, an exchange for not being the primary breadwinner.

Within these definitions, several features are important. It is recognized that everyone requires or needs care, not just those we consider incapable of caring for themselves by reason of age, disability, or illness. Often, only children, the elderly, the disabled, and the chronically ill are seen as requiring care, while the need for care and receiving of care by so-called independent adults is suppressed or denied. As Sara Ruddick notes, "most recipients of care are only partially 'dependent' and often becoming less so; most of their 'needs', even those clearly physical cannot be separated from more elusive emotional requirements for respect, affection, and cheer."[2] At the same time, even those individuals we see as fully independent, that is, able to care for themselves in terms of "activities of daily living," may for reasons of time or energy, or temporary condition, need or desire care to maintain their physical, psychological, and emotional well-being. They may turn to a family member, friends, a servant, or a service provider for hot meals, physical touch, or a sympathetic ear. The difference is that independent adults may preserve their sense of independence if they have sufficient economic or social resources, so as to command care from others rather than being beholden to relatives or charity.

Another aspect is that care is seen as creating a relationship; as Sara Ruddick puts it, "[caring] work is constituted in and through the relationship of those who give and receive care." The relationship is one of interdependence. Generally we think of the caregiver as having the power in the relationship, but the care receiver, even if subordinate or dependent, also has agency and even power in the relationship. Focusing on relationships brings into relief the influence of the recipients of care on caring work. Tronto notes that for the work of care to be successful, its recipients have to respond appropriately (e.g., a screaming child or a moaning elderly person betokens failure). In some situations, where the care receiver employs the caregiver (and therefore controls wages and working conditions) or has social authority (e.g., from the norm of respect toward elders), the care receiver may have more power than the caregiver.[3]

We must also recognize that caring is organized in myriad ways. The paradigmatic care relationship is that between mother and child, which often serves as the template for thinking about caring. In this model, caring (mothering) is viewed as natural and instinctive and as women's natural vocation. However, this idealized model is deceptive in that it ignores the actual diversity in the ways mothering/caring is actually carried out within and across cultures. Caring can and does take place in the household or in publicly organized institutions and can be carried out individually or collectively, as paid or unpaid labor. Much caring takes place in the family, usually as the unpaid work of women, but it is also done as paid work (e.g., by babysitters or home health aides). It also takes place in the community as unpaid volunteer work, as in the case of church or charitable organizations that run day-care or senior activity centers. It also takes place in institutions organized by the state, corporations, or individuals as commodified services using paid caregivers.

Care can also be "fragmented," that is, divided among several caregivers and between "private" and "public" settings. Thus a parent may take ultimate responsibility for ensuring that a child has care after school but delegate the actual work of caregiving to a babysitter, a relative, a paid homecare worker, and/or an after-school program. Barrie Thorne found in her study of childhoods in an urban multicultural community that parents often have to patch together several of these arrangements.[4]

What Should Be Our Goals?

To achieve a society in which caring work is valued in all spheres of social life, all of the elements—the caring relationship, the work of caregiving, and the people involved (care receivers, and caregivers)— should be recognized and valued. Hence a society in which caring is valued would be one in which:

- Caring is recognized as "real work" and as a social contribution on a par with other activities that are valued, such as paid employment, military service, or community service, regardless of whether caring takes place in the family or elsewhere or as paid or unpaid labor.
- Those who need or require care (including children, the elderly, disabled, and chronically ill) are recognized as full members of the society and accorded corresponding rights, social standing, and voice. This would mean that care receivers are empowered to have influence over the type of care, the setting, and the caretaker,

and that they have access to sufficient material resources to obtain adequate care.

- Those who do caring work are accorded social recognition and entitlements for their efforts similar to those who contribute through other forms of work or other activities. These entitlements include working conditions and supports that enable them to do their work well and an appropriate level of economic return, whether in wages or social entitlements.

For these ideals to be achieved, certain conditions need to be honored:

- Caring is recognized as a community and collective (public) responsibility rather than as purely a family (private) responsibility.
- Access to care and to "high-quality" care is relatively equally distributed and not dependent on economic or social status. Ultimately the ideal would be a society in which there is an adequate amount and quality of care for all who need it, (i.e., care that is individualized, culturally appropriate, and responsive to the preferences of those who are cared for). A similar goal involving access to medical care for all members of society has gained substantial political support.
- The responsibility and actual work of caring are relatively equitably shared so that the burden of care does not fall disproportionately, as it does now, on disadvantaged groups—women, racialized minorities, and immigrants.

Why is the goal of achieving a society that values caring and caring relationships important? It seems inherent in the definition of a good society that those who cannot care for themselves are cared for, that people can trust that if they become dependent, they will be cared for, and that they feel able to care for those they care about. Additionally, valuing care and caring relationships would contribute to building a more just society. Because caregiving is disproportionately carried out by women and by people of color, the devaluing of caring contributes to the marginalization, exploitation, and dependency of these groups. Conversely, valuing and recognizing caring and caring relationships would expand the boundaries of equality to many currently excluded from social equality.

Although these goals and aspirations might appear almost utopian to Americans, in fact they are not. A number of European countries—such as the Netherlands, Norway, and Denmark—no more economically advanced than the United States—have chosen precisely these societal goals and have moved dramatically toward achieving them. Thus, we know that the objectives are not really utopian; they merely require leadership and commitment.

Some Directions for Change

One important change would be to redefine "social citizenship" to make care central to the rights and entitlements of citizens. This will involve a reversal of the present situation where care is defined as a private responsibility and therefore outside the realm of citizenship. Making care central to citizenship will entail three elements: establishing a right to care as a core right of citizens, establishing caregiving as a public social responsibility, and according caregivers recognition for carrying out a public social responsibility. These elements are interrelated. If citizens have a right to receive care, then there is a corresponding responsibility on the part of the community to ensure that those who need care get it. Further, if caregiving is a public social responsibility, then those who perform caregiving fulfill an obligation of citizenship and are thus entitled to societal benefits comparable to those accorded to those fulfilling the obligation to earn (for example, social security, seniority, and retirement benefits).

There are some additional considerations, however, because of the gendered organization of caring and the "secondary dependence" of unpaid caretakers who forgo earning to undertake care. Joan Tronto warns that policies have to be carefully crafted so as not to recreate gender inequities in caring. Cancian and Oliker, reworking Barbara Hobson's concepts of citizen worker and citizen mother, identify several types of welfare policies: carer citizen, worker citizen, and carer-worker citizen.[5]

Worker citizen policies provide entitlements for breadwinners and their dependents through programs such as unemployment insurance and survivor benefits. These policies encourage men, who are generally able to earn more than women, to specialize in earning and women to focus on unpaid caregiving. Worker citizen policies exist in many countries, but it is the principal approach used by the U.S. welfare system.[6]

In most European countries carer citizen policies complement worker citizen policies by providing direct benefits to caregivers through programs such as mother's allowances and caregiver pensions. Carer citizen policies reinforce the gender division of earning versus caring by encouraging women to specialize in caring. However, it also supports them for doing so through payments and services that are treated as entitlements and are not means tested.

Carer-worker citizen policies provide supports and benefits for citizens who combine caring and earning through such programs as paid parental leave, employment-based child care, and the crediting of years spent in caring and in earning equally toward retirement. Such policies are most prevalent in Scandinavian welfare systems. Cancian and Oliker note that carer-worker policies "are least likely to reinforce full-time caregiving for women and are most supportive of women and men sharing earning and caring." Carer-worker policies have not succeeded in degendering caring work, but they have encouraged some shifting. For example, Norway's parental leave policy, which sets aside a portion of total leave that can only be taken by fathers, has encouraged men's involvement in caring.[7]

An additional constraint that is specific to caring (in contrast to earning) and that needs to be addressed is what Eva Kittay has called the "secondary dependence" of the caregiver. By taking on the care of a dependent and forgoing earning, unpaid caregivers become dependent on a third party—a breadwinner or the state—for resources to sustain both those they care for (primary dependents) and themselves (secondary dependents).[8] Historically, U.S. welfare policy has been premised on the assumption that support for caregiving belonged to the male breadwinner and that the state should assume responsibility for support of caring only in the absence of a male breadwinner. Sometimes, as in the case of black single mothers, the absence of a male breadwinner was not seen as calling for the state to step in. Instead, black single mothers were deemed to be "employable mothers" who should support themselves and their dependents. As described earlier, in a step backward from recognizing caregivers' need for support, the U.S. Congress passed the Personal Responsibility and Work Opportunity Reconciliation Act in 1996, which replaced the Aid to Families with Dependent

Children program with Temporary Assistance to Needy Families. As a result, poor mothers are restricted to only five years of benefits during their entire lifetimes, regardless of need, and are required by most states to meet various stringent employment requirements.

In contrast to the U.S. welfare system, European welfare systems have all provided some forms of family allowance for citizens with children. Most countries support caregivers with child allowances, and some even give small pensions for those who engage in unpaid care work. In countries with relatively conservative welfare regimes, such as France and Germany, the rationale for maternal allowances typically has been framed in terms of child welfare and promoting natalism, so as to ensure the size and well-being of the future population, rather than in terms of the value of caring and social citizenship rights and responsibilities in caring. Nonetheless, the allowances have been designed as universal entitlements not tied to income or means testing, unlike U.S. welfare programs. In more progressive social democratic countries, such as Sweden, support for caregiving is extensive, including allowances, subsidies, and direct services such as childcare and home aides.[9]

In short, what is called for is a three-pronged expansion of social citizenship rights to: (1) make caretaking allowances and support universal (as in the case of Social Security) rather than being means tested; (2) have such support explicitly framed as entitlements for carrying out an important citizenship responsibility, not as charity or replacement of a breadwinner's contribution; and (3) provide support for combining employment/earning and caregiving, so as to equalize the costs and benefits of caregiving versus earning. The latter feature is important so as not to penalize women for caregiving and also to avoid reinforcing the gender division of labor in which men earn and women care.

Transforming social citizenship in the United States to make care central to rights and entitlements would require a challenge to the linked ideologies of individual independence and family responsibility. The United States for the most part has not even recognized caring as a contribution to the national welfare, nor has it assumed a larger societal responsibility for supporting caregivers. As with previous changes in the boundaries and meanings of citizenship, this one would require a concerted struggle; political citizenship, in the form of suffrage, was gradually expanded to include previously excluded groups such as nonpropertied white men in the early nineteenth century, black men after the Civil War, and finally women in 1920. The expansion of the right to vote was achieved only after organized campaigns waged by each of the excluded groups over the course of over 100 years. Similarly, social citizenship rights such as social security, unemployment relief, minimum wage, and job creation were responses to the political mobilization of millions of Americans displaced by the Great Depression.[10] In the second half of the twentieth century, the second civil rights movement and second-wave feminism impelled legal, political, and social changes that dramatically expanded employment, education, and legal rights for racial minorities and women.

An important example of expanding citizenship is the success of the disability rights movement in establishing federal laws and policies that require schools and universities, employers, and public entities to provide facilities and programs that enable differently abled citizens to work, study, travel, and otherwise participate in the social and cultural life of the society. The disability rights movement comes quite close to addressing the issues central to caring and social citizenship. It focuses on the rights of citizens who have physical and mental conditions that limit their physical and economic independence to receive services and accommodations that allow them to achieve social and political independence.[11] There is thus a precedent for claiming the right to *receive* care as essential for meaningful citizenship. What is more difficult is to make the case for rights and entitlements for those *providing* care.

Another change is to rethink the family as the primary site of care. U.S. policies on social citizenship and care have assumed that most care takes place within the family and is carried out as part of unpaid labor by family members. However, if we take seriously the notion that caring is a public responsibility, we need to critically examine the idea of the family as the institution of first resort for caring. Indeed, one can argue that keeping the family as the "natural" unit for caring relationships helps to anchor the gender division of caring labor. Seeing family and women's caring as "natural" disguises the material relationships of dependence that undergird the arrangement. Love is not enough; care requires material resources. We need to consider ways to free women from disproportionate responsibility for caregiving and also to free both care receivers and caregivers from economic dependency.

There have been some successful movements to create small-scale "intentional communities," often formed around some commonality such as religion, ecological concerns, vegetarianism, interest in higher education, or sexual orientation, in which people can socialize, share meals and chores, and assist one another. These communities are premised on governance by the residents themselves. Some intentional communities are multigenerational, but a growing number are made up of those in their "golden years" who wish to age in place. One form of intentional community is co-housing, a concept borrowed from Denmark, in which families or individuals have individual housing units clustered around a common building in which neighbors can gather for meals, meetings, or watching television together. Residents make decisions about maintenance and other management matters collectively. Another form is created through a non-profit organization that enrolls members who pay yearly dues. The community that is created operates as a "one-stop" entity for services and programs ranging from social and cultural events to transportation and home maintenance and arranging for home care from a designated provider. Beacon Hill Village in Boston and Capital Hill Village in Washington, D.C. are examples of this model. As the word "village" in the names conveys, these organizations invoke the rural settlements of the past in which neighbors knew, cared about, and willingly helped one another in times of need. In the urban settings in which they are located, these organizations rely on volunteer forces and employ the internet to build community, encourage mutual assistance, and coordinate access to resources. Intentional communities represent a more collective approach to care but at present are available to a relatively small segment of the population, generally more affluent people who can choose their living situations.[12]

For both practical and ideological reasons it seems likely that the family (broadly defined) will remain a primary institution for providing care for children and, to a lesser extent, for the elderly and the disabled. However, this does not mean that the family should be defined in the traditional way as a conjugal heterosexual household or that it should be the first resort for care in all cases. The official care policies of state and federal entities as well as those of corporate employers currently recognize dependency and caring relationships in rather traditional terms of parents and children (whether biological or adoptive) and spouses (defined through legal marriage or legally registered domestic partnerships). The fact is that in the United States the reality of how a "family" is organized and constituted, who is in it, and how it functions has changed dramatically since World War II. There are many types of family relations that generate relationships of care, including extended kin such as grandparents and siblings, cohabiting couples (heterosexual or gay and lesbian), and sometimes "fictive kin." As Carol Stack and Linda Burton point out in relation to their study of African American families, men, women, and children may be "kin-scripted" to care for nieces and nephews, grandparents, grandchildren, and aunts and uncles when there is no one else capable of doing so. To the extent that caring in the "family" is valued, the notion of "family" has to be extended to encompass diverse kin relations, including "voluntary" or "fictive" relationships.[13]

Regarding the knotty question of the primacy of family versus larger community in caregiving, in a survey conducted in England by Janet Finch, respondents affirmed the importance of kin ties; they indicated that "rallying around in times of crisis" was what defined a functional family. The actual degree of responsibility that respondents felt in particular situations and toward particular relatives varied, however, depending on prior relationship and current circumstances. In general, Finch's respondents emphasized that relatives should not expect or take for granted assistance from other family members. Another British researcher, Jenny Morris, interviewed disabled adult women, many of whom said they preferred paid helpers or helpers provided by social service to help from family members because it allowed them more independence. Some disabled women said that they preferred helpers they paid themselves over those paid by the state because it gave them more control over the care they received.[14]

Finch argues that the moral reasoning of people in her survey suggests the principle that people should have the right not to have to rely on their families for help: "To point in another way, the family should not be seen as the option of first resort for giving assistance to its adult members, either financial or practical." Finch is careful to say that her point is not to deprecate generosity, care, and support within families but only to see these as "optional, voluntary, freely given."[15] The implication of Finch's argument is that public policy should assume that everyone is entitled to publicly organized care regardless of whether or not family members are available to provide care.

Taken together, the findings from Finch's and Morris's studies support the case that the community, as represented by the state, has primary responsibility for care of its citizens and that citizens in turn have the right to non-family care. Under such a system, it is more likely that family members who do undertake care will be doing so voluntarily and freely and makes it clearer that they are undertaking work that contributes to the public and not just private good. Thus adopting the principle that the community or the state, not the family, should be the first resort in caring would reinforce the principle that family caregivers deserve and require economic support and services. As we have seen, many programs for disabled and elderly people already exist at the state and federal level to provide payments and other support for family caregivers. This provision should be made universal under federal Medicare.

Another approach is rethinking paid care. The sheer demand for care as a result of the expansion of the elderly population, the inability of families to provide all the care needed, and the availability of government-funded allowances through Medicaid have brought about an unprecedented growth in paid caregiving. A significant portion of marketized care work takes place in institutional settings, assisted-living facilities, nursing homes, hospitals, and residential facilities, where the intensive face-to-face caring is done by nursing aides and other non-professional workers under the supervision of administrators and medical and nursing professionals. This is especially the case for those needing physically demanding around-the-clock care, such as children and adults with severe mental and physical disabilities and the elderly with advanced dementia or Alzheimer's. Nonetheless, the overall trend has been to keep dependents out of institutions by caring for them at home, so a great deal of marketized care is done in private households by home-care workers employed by non-profit or for-profit agencies or by care recipients themselves (or their relatives).

The biggest issue raised by marketized care is whether economic motives and caring motives are compatible. Returning to our earlier definition of caring work as involving on the one hand "caring activities" and on the other hand "caring feelings," we can ask whether, when people are paid for caring, they focus on caring activities and give short shrift to caring feelings. Marketized care has been decried by people on both the left and the right. On the left, there is suspicion of capitalism and its tendency to turn everything into a commodity, so that care becomes an impersonal "product," produced at least cost and sold to the highest bidder to generate profit.[16] On the right, social conservatives exalt traditional "family values," see family care as invariably superior, and want to preserve the private household as a protected sphere of altruism and love. We have seen that there has been considerable resistance to allowing those eligible for Medicare-funded home care services to hire and pay relatives. The concern is that being paid would erode the sense of family responsibility. Spouses, parents, and children would be providing care for the "wrong reasons," or perhaps relatives who would otherwise be unwilling to provide care for free would take on care for monetary reasons. In either case, it is feared that the quality of care would suffer.

This reasoning assumes a dichotomy between paid and unpaid work: that those who work for money are motivated purely by materialism, self-interest, and greed, whereas those who work without pay are motivated by altruism, spiritual values, and affection. In short, it assumes that people work either for money or for love. However, as we have seen in the preceding chapters, there are many more complex meanings and intentions involved in monetary exchanges other than materialism, for instance, a parent paying child support based on concern for the child and not as an economic exchange. In a similar fashion, allowances or wages for caring for family members can be viewed as acknowledgement of the loving care they provide, not as a "bribe" to do what they would not otherwise do. Thus family caregivers who receive admittedly meager payments from disabled or elderly programs look at the pay they receive not as a quid pro quo but as social recognition and validation of their contributions. (The amount in any case is not enough to support them fully but enables them to contribute to their own support and to get by with additional assistance from other family members.)

Similarly, work for pay involves more than material self-interest or greed. The working man is assumed to be an independent and self-interested actor in the market. However, a married working man is commended as "breadwinner" for providing for the needs of his wife and children. Indeed, the argument that working men are breadwinners was used historically to argue for a family wage for men. The notion of the male breadwinner acknowledges that as a worker he is not acting strictly as an autonomous individual but as a connected human being enmeshed in social relations and concerned about his family's well-being. Ideally, the breadwinner is acting altruistically when he shares/uses his earnings to provide for his wife's and children's maintenance.

Working for pay does not therefore necessarily negate the intrinsic aspects of work. Philosopher Margaret Radin makes a distinction between the "laborer," who is motivated solely by money and thus experiences labor as separate from the real self, and the "worker," for whom work has a more complex meaning. She notes, "Workers make money but are also at the same time givers. Money does not fully motivate them to work, nor does it exhaust the value of their activity. Work is understood not as separate from life and self, but rather as a part of the worker, and indeed constitutive of her. Nor is work understood as separate from relations with other people."[17]

I don't want to make the distinction between work and labor in the way Radin does; however, I do want to hold on to the idea that there is a range of orientations that workers can have toward work that go beyond that of economic exchange. This idea, that paid workers have non-economic orientations, complements the earlier stated idea that family carers retain their "intrinsic" (non-economic) motivation to care even when they are compensated monetarily for their care. Too often, low wages for care workers are rationalized on the grounds that care work offers intrinsic rewards that compensate for lack of material rewards or even, especially in the case of family caregivers, that too much monetary compensation would undermine altruistic feelings.

Thus, any scheme to create a society in which caring is valued in all spheres of society must address the growing commodification of care. We need to think about the implications of changes that take place in caring work when "strangers" rather than family members provide care, when it is paid rather than unpaid, and, most importantly, when it is regulated and controlled by impersonal rules and hierarchy.

Deborah Stone found that home-care workers faced a conflict between bureaucratic rules and their own ethic of care. Workers reported that they often stretched rules or evaded supervisors in order to provide personal care; some said they spent off-work time or money to provide extra services.[18] Giving workers latitude to attend to social and emotional aspects of care would increase the intrinsic rewards of the job. Because direct care workers are in a position to assess first hand what the needs of the care recipient are, empowering them to take initiatives in shaping services would also be salutary.

At the same time, empowering caregivers without also empowering care recipients poses the risk of exacerbating the already unequal relationships between caregivers and care receivers. Caregivers may feel that they understand the needs of care receivers and that they are acting in their best interests. However, care receivers might have different values and priorities. To the extent that care receivers are emotionally and physically dependent on their caregivers, they may feel they have no choice but to defer to the caregiver's judgment.

Thus an additional concern should be to ensure that care receivers are given voice and influence over their care. Mentally competent adults requiring home-care assistance, for example, might be given grants to hire their own caregivers rather than being assigned a helper by a social service agency. One of the 50 disabled women interviewed by Jenny Morris in England said that only when she started employing her own helper did she feel she could pay attention to her own appearance. She had her paid helper assist her with clothing and makeup, which she felt justified in doing because "They need to be patient and I'm paying for that patience so I feel OK about expecting it."[19] In the United States, one major group already has direct access to government grants with which to hire care workers. The Department of Veterans Affairs has a program called Universal Aid and Attendance Allowance that gives direct unrestricted cash payments to 220,000 veterans to pay for homecare workers or "attendants."[20] The right of veterans to be paid for hiring their own care workers is acknowledged because of their service to the country. What is needed is a more universal approach that extends the right to non-familial paid care for all categories of citizens.[21]

In short, both paid caregivers and receivers of paid care need to be empowered. Sometimes, when the interests of caregivers and care recipients intersect, it makes sense for them to organize together. For example, when social service agency budgets are cut and home care and other services are reduced, caregivers may be forced to serve more clients less well, and clients do not get the care they need. During the 1980s and 1990s, home health-care workers and receivers and community leaders joined together to form coalitions to press for better wages and benefits for care workers. Because services are paid from Medicaid and other public funds, care receivers have good reason to support wage increases for care workers, especially if it means that their caregivers will continue providing care rather than leave for higher paying jobs in other fields.[22] However, as funding crises in many states in the 2008–2010 period have shown, state budget cuts are imposed most dramatically on the politically weakest sectors, especially the elderly and disabled. The case of California, where prison funding survived largely intact in part because of pressures from prison guard unions, while home care programs for the elderly and disabled were severely cut, emphasizes the importance of organization and political clout.

We also need to change employment practices to make it possible for people to integrate work and care so that caregiving is not penalized. A small proportion of citizens currently benefit from private-sector initiatives by corporations that recognize the caring responsibilities of their employees. Some of these employers provide child care and leaves to care for children or elderly relatives. Model programs have included those by Citibank, Stride Rite, and Campbell's Soups, which provided child care on or near their premises. Bristol Myers-Squibb initiated a family leave policy for employees that covered care for elderly relatives.[23]

The passage of the 1993 Family and Medical Leave Act marked a first step in developing a national policy in support of combining work and care. The act recognized care responsibilities for those engaged in paid work and accepted public responsibility for dependents receiving adequate care. As in many European countries, the stated goal of the legislation was enhancement of children and the family unit rather than recognition of caregiving as a larger social responsibility. The act's preamble recognized job security and parenting as important for citizens' well-being and acknowledged the role of the state in supporting both. However, coverage was extremely limited. By requiring only unpaid leave, the government only accommodates care rather than supporting it because few parents can afford to make use of the unpaid leave. Moreover, by exempting employers with fewer than 50 employees it left out about half of the U.S. workforce; 56 percent of women and 48 percent of men were not covered. Finally, the act recognized dependency only within traditional conjugal family relationships: spouse, children, and parents.[24] It thereby narrowly defined the now-mythological "family unit" in which care occurs and excluded the many other real-world relationships in which dependency and care actually exist.

In addition to parental and caretaking leave and child-care provisions, employment policy needs to take into account the sheer number of hours needed for care. A 1999 national survey of 1,509 English-speaking households in the United States found an average of 17.9 hours of caregiving per week per household, and several other specialized surveys have found a much higher number of unpaid caregivers in households with persons having special medical conditions or disabilities.[25] Simultaneously, the work hours of employed Americans are among the longest in industrialized countries. A 2007 survey of work hours by the Organization for Economic Cooperation and Development found that U.S. workers worked more hours per year than those in almost every other industrial nation, including Japan. The difference between Americans and Europeans was particularly striking, with Norwegian and Dutch workers putting in 25 percent fewer hours and Germans working 20 percent and French 15 percent fewer hours.[26]

In combination with lack of state support for caregivers, long hours increase the strain on U.S. workers who have care responsibilities. Comparisons of worker productivity suggest that the longer hours of U.S. workers have not resulted in comparable increases in productivity. Thus reduction of work hours can be justified on economic as well as social welfare grounds. The 40-hour week was the goal of labor movements starting after the Civil War, but it was only when organized labor acquired sufficient political power in the 1930s that it became the standard. It involved the recognition of workers' rights for a life apart from the job. It is now time to recognize the reality of workers' multiple responsibilities for earning and caring by including caring work in the overall equation.

Finally, it needs to be said that inequalities between men and women in the labor market help to maintain gendered caring. The use of anti-discrimination law, affirmative-action policies, and comparable-worth strategies to promote gender equality in the labor market would contribute toward more equitable division of caring by making it equally attractive or costly for men and women to forego earning to engage in caring.[27]

Achieving the kinds of changes needed to produce a society that values caring will require transforming the ways we think about ourselves, our relationships with others, the family, civil society, the state, and the political economy. Ultimately the transformation of caring must be linked to changes in political economic structures and relationships. Perhaps most fundamentally, the concept of "society" as made up of discrete, independent, and freely choosing individuals will have to become more accurate and realistic. We must understand that interdependence among not wholly autonomous members of society is occurring because of the unquestioned demographic trajectories of the twenty-first century that are leading to larger numbers of elderly and others in need of care. The recent history of the United States and of advanced democracies in Europe has shown that such changes are achievable, and that they can lead to more just societies in which all individuals—regardless of age, gender, race, or beliefs—can lead more fulfilling lives.

Notes

1. Who Cares?

1. U.S. Census Bureau, Population Data Division, International Data Base, "Population Pyramid Summary for United States," available at http://docs .google.com/viewer?a=v&q=cache:qcEYHJhoVwMJ:www.charlottediocese .org/customers/101092709242178/filemanager/docmgr/pyramid_usa.pdf (accessed December 8, 2009).
2. Mona Harrington, *Care and Equality: Inventing a New Family Politics* (New York: Knopf, 1999), 17.
3. Bureau of Labor Statistics, U.S. Department of Labor, *Women in the Labor Force: A Data Book* (Washington, DC: Government Printing Office, 2008), 1.
4. International Labour Organization, *Key Indicators of the Labour Market*, 5th ed. (Geneva: Brookings Institute Press, 2008), figure 6b, available at http://www.ilo.org/empelm/what/pubs/lang–en/WCMS_114060/index .htm (accessed January 3, 2009).
5. Arlie Russell Hochschild, *The Time Bind: When Work Becomes Home and Home Becomes Work* (New York: Holt, 1997).
6. Suzanna D. Smith, "What Is Caregiving?" Fact Sheet FCS 2082, Department of Family, Youth and Community Sciences, Florida Cooperative Extension Service, Institute of Food and Agricultural Sciences, University of Florida 1999, rev. 2005, 2, PDF document available at http://edis.ifas.ufl .edu/HE017 (accessed December 1, 2008).
7. Ibid.
8. National Alliance for Caregiving and AARP, *Caregiving in the U.S.: A Focused Look at Those Caring for Someone 50 or Older* (2009), 14, 34, PDF version available at http://www.aarp.org/research/surveys/care/ltc/hc/articles/ caregiving_09.html (accessed December 10, 2009).
9. A study issued by the U.S. Department of Health and Human Services, *Informal Caregiving: Compassion in Action* (Washington, DC, 1998), 18, estimated that three-fourths of primary informal caregivers of elderly were women; The National Alliance for Caregiving and AARP study, *Caregiving in the U.S.,* reported that 67 percent of those caring for adults 50 or older

were women. An earlier survey study by the National Alliance for Caregiving and AARP, *Caregiving in the U.S.* (2004), 8, found that women caregivers provided an average of four more hours a week of care than their male counterparts and made up 71 percent of those caring for those requiring the highest level of care. The downloadable report is available at http://www.caregiving.org/data/04finalreport.pdf (accessed December 18, 2009).

10. U.S. Department of Health and Human Services, *Informal Caregiving*, 8.

11. Pamela Doty, Mary E. Jackson, and William Crown, "The Impact of Female Caregivers' Employment Status on Patterns of Formal and Informal Eldercare," *The Gerontologist* 38, no. 3 (1998): 335, table 2.

12. Data collected for *Caregiving in the U.S.* (2009), 28, found that 68 percent of African American caregivers said they had been employed during some period when they were giving care compared to 56 percent of white caregivers.

13. The *Caregiving in the U.S.* survey (2009) found the average age of caregivers was 46 (p. 2).

14. Charles R. Pierret, "The 'Sandwich Generation': Women Caring for Parents and Children," *Monthly Labor Review* (September 2006): 3–9, found that, depending on definition (co-residence, amount of financial support, hours of assistance), between 9 percent and 33 percent of 45- to 56-year-old women fall into the sandwich generation.

15. MetLife Mature Market Institute, National Alliance for Caregiving (NAC), and National Center on Women and Aging, *The MetLife Juggling Act Study: Balancing Caregiving with Work and the Costs Involved* (New York: Metlife Mature Market Institute, 1999), 3, PDF document available at http://www.metlife.com/mmi/publications/research-studies/index.html (accessed January 21, 2009).

16. Peter P. Vitaliano, Jianping Zhang, and James M. Scanlan, "Is Caregiving Hazardous to One's Physical Health? A Meta-Analysis," *Psychological Bulletin* 129, no. 6 (2003): 946–972, analyzes the combined findings of 23 studies. See also Family Caregiver Alliance, "Fact Sheet: Caregiver Health," available at http://www.caregiver.org/caregiver/jsp/content_node.jsp?nodeid=1822 (accessed December 18, 2009), which summarizes findings from several score of studies.

17. National Alliance for Caregiving and AARP, *Caregiving in the U.S.* (2009), 35.

18. MetLife Mature Market Institute, National Alliance for Caregiving (NAC), and National Center on Women and Aging, *The MetLife Juggling Act Study*, 5, 6.

19. Chizuko Wakabayashi and Katharine M. Donato, "Caregiving for Economic Well-Being in Women's Later Life," *Journal of Health and Social Behavior* 47, no. 3 (2006): 258–274.

20. Richard W. Johnson and Joshua M. Wiener, "A Profile of Frail Older Americans and Their Caregivers," Occasional Paper Number 8, The Retirement Project (Washington, DC: Urban Institute, 2006), figure 4.2, 24.

21. William J. Scanlon, *Nursing Workforce: Recruitment and Retention of Nurses and Nurse Aides Is a Growing Concern,* Statement to Committee on Health, Education, Labor, and Pensions, U.S. Senate (Washington, DC: U.S. General Accounting Office, May 17, 2001); Maureen Mickus, Claire C. Luz, and Andrew Hogan, *Voices from the Front: Recruitment and Retention of Direct Care Workers in Long Term Care across Michigan* (East Lansing: Michigan State University, April 22, 2004), available at http://www.directcare clearinghouse.org/download/MI_vocices_from_the_front.pdf (accessed January 27, 2009).

22. U.S. Bureau of Labor Statistics, *Career Guide to Industries, 2008–09 Edition: Health Care,* calculated from table 2, available at http://www.bls.gov/oco/cg/cgs035.htm (accessed January 16, 2009).

23. Paraprofessional Healthcare Institute, *State Chart Book on Wages for Personal and Home Care Aides, 1999–2008* (San Francisco: Center for Personal Assistance Services, University of California, San Francisco, 2008), 4, available at http://www.pascenter.org/publications/publication_home.php?id=979 (accessed December 8, 2009).

24. Sophie Korczyk, *Long-Term Workers in Five Countries: Issues and Options* (Washington, DC: AARP Public Policy Institute, 2004), 7.

25. Mickus, Luz, and Hogan, *Voices from the Front,* 25, figure 5; Bureau of Labor Statistics, U.S. Department of Labor, "Injuries to Caregivers Working in Patients' Homes," *Issues in Labor Statistics* 97, no. 4 (February 1997), available at http://www.bls.gov/opub/ils/pdf/opbils11.pdf (accessed December 12, 2009).

26. Rhonda J. V. Montgomery, Lyn Holley, Jerome Deichert, and Karl Kosloski, "A Profile of Home Care Workers from the 2000 Census: How It Changes What We Know," *Gerontologist* 45 (2005): 593–600.

27. Candace Howes, "Love, Money, or Flexibility: What Motivates People to Work in Consumer-Directed Home Care?" *The Gerontologist* 48 (2008): 46–60.

28. Montgomery et al., "A Profile of Home Care Workers."

29. Candace Howes, "Building a High Quality Home Care Workforce: Wages, Benefits and Flexibility Matter," Better Jobs Better Care, Institute for the Future of Aging Services, American Association of Home Services for Aging, available at 87 (accessed December 12, 2009).

30. Mickus, Luz, and Hogan, *Voices from the Front;* Robyn I. Stone, "The Direct Care Worker: The Third Rail of Home Care Policy," *Annual Review of Public Health* 25 (2004): 521–537.

31. Micaela DiLeonardo, "The Female World of Cards and Holidays: Women, Families and the Work of Kinship," *Signs* 12, no. 3 (1987): 440–453; Cheryl Townsend Gilkes, *If It Wasn't for the Women: Black Women's Experience and Womanist Culture in Church and Community* (Maryknoll, NY: Orbis Books, 2001), 61–75.

32. Alvin Gouldner, "The Norm of Reciprocity: A Preliminary Statement," *American Sociological Review* 25, no. 2 (April 1960): 170.

33. Henry Sumner Maine, *Ancient Law* (Sioux Falls, SD: NuVision Publications, 2009; orig. 1861), 70; Amy Dru Stanley, *From Bondage to Contract: Wage Labor, Marriage, and the Market in the Age of Slave Emancipation* (Cambridge: Cambridge University Press, 1998), 1–2.

2. Caring for One's Own and Caring for a Living

1. The terms "production" and "reproduction," adopted by (Marxist feminist) scholars, originated in Friedrich Engels's remark that the "determining factor in history is, in the final instance, the production and reproduction of immediate life. This . . . is of a twofold character: on the one side, the production of the means of existence, of food, clothing and shelter and the tools necessary for that production; on the other side, the production of human beings themselves, the propagation of the species." Friedrich Engels, *The Origin of the Family, Private Property and the State* (New York: International Publishers, 1972), 71. I use the terms "reproduction" and "social reproduction" more or less interchangeably with "care labor" in that they all refer to the work required to maintain people as social, emotional, and intellectual beings on a daily and intergenerational basis.

2. Mary Ann Mason, *From Father's Property to Children's Rights: A History of Child Custody* (New York: Columbia University Press, 1994), 6; Alice Kessler-Harris, *Out to Work: A History of Wage- Earning Women in the United States* (New York: Oxford University Press, 1982), 7; John Demos, *A Little Commonwealth: Family Life in Plymouth Colony,* 2nd ed. (New York: Oxford University Press, 1999), 100–106; Carl Degler, *At Odds: Women and the Family from the Revolution to the Present* (New York: Oxford University Press 1980), 363–367.

3. Laurel Thatcher Ulrich, *Good Wives: Image and Reality in the Lives of Women in Northern New England, 1650–1750* (New York: Oxford University Press, 1983), 35–49; Lisa Norling, "Judith Macy and Her DayBook; or, Crevecoeur and the Wives of Sherborn," *Historic Nantucket* 40, no. 4 (Winter 1992): 70–71. Kirsten E. Wood, in "Broken Reeds and Competent Farmers: Slaveholding Widows in the Southeastern United States, 1783–1861," *Journal of Women's History* 13, no. 2 (Summer 2001): 47, notes a similar position for southern wives of being "doubles" for their husbands.

4. Susan Branson, "Women and the Family Economy in the Early Republic: The Case of Elizabeth Meredith," *Journal of the Early Republic* 16, no. 1 (Spring 1996): 52; Ellen Hartigan-O'Connor, "'She Said She Did Not Know Money:' Urban Women and Atlantic Markets in the Revolutionary Era," *Early American Studies* 4, no. 2 (Fall 2006): 322–352; Serena Zabin, "Women's Trading Networks and Dangerous Economies in Eighteenth Century New York City," *Early American Studies* 4, no. 2 (Fall 2006): 291–321; Gerda Lerner, "The Lady and the Mill Girl: Changes in the Status of Women in the Age of Jackson," *Midcontinent American Studies Journal* 10, no. 1 (Spring 1969): 5–15; Claudia Goldin, "The Economic Status of Women in the Early Republic: Quantitative Evidence," *Journal of Interdisciplinary History* 16, no. 3 (Winter 1986): 375–404.

5. Lerner, "The Lady and the Mill Girl," 5–15; Goldin, "The Economic Status of Women," 375–404.

6. Nancy Fraser and Linda Gordon, "A Genealogy of *Dependency:* Tracing a Key Word in the U.S. Welfare State," *Signs* 19, no. 2 (1994): 313.

7. Chilton Williamson, *American Suffrage: From Property to Democracy, 1760–1860* (Princeton, NJ: Princeton University Press, 1960), 104; Philip Foner, *History of Black Americans,* vol. 1: *From Africa to the Emergence of the Cotton Kingdom* (Westport, CT: Greenwood Press, 1975), 517–518; Joan R. Gunderson, "Independence, Citizenship, and the American Revolution," *Signs* 13, no. 1 (1987): 66.

8. William E. Forbath, "Caste, Class, and Second-Class Citizenship," *Michigan Law Review* 98 (October 1999): 20.

9. Rosemarie Zagarri, "The Rights of Man and Woman in Post-Revolutionary America," *William and Mary Quarterly* 55, no. 2 (April 1998): 213.

10. Ibid., 221.

11. Ibid., 224.

12. J. G. A. Pocock, "The Ideal of Citizenship since Classical Times," in Ronald Beiner, ed., *Theorizing Citizenship* (Albany: State University of New York Press, 1995), 30–32.

13. Linda K. Kerber, *Women of the Republic: Intellect and Ideology in Revolutionary America* (Chapel Hill: University of North Carolina Press, 1980).

14. Joan R. Gunderson, *To Be Useful to the World: Women in Revolutionary America, 1740–1790* (New York: Twayne Publishers, 1996), 172, 173. One could also say there was a notion of Republican womanhood, since women also had duties as Republican wives: "If virtue was to check power, women would have to civilize men and teach them virtue. For women the way to serve the public was to purify their lives and pray for the community" (p. 173).

15. Ibid., 173.

16. Ibid., 181.

17. Ibid., 179.

18. John Lauritz Larson, "The Market Revolution in Early America: An Introduction," *OAH Magazine of History* (May 2005): 4. The term "market revolution" is often used loosely to refer to a host of economic developments
preceding the full-blown industrialization in the post–Civil War years. Its
periodization is also subject to debate, with some historians describing
its emergence in the latter part of the eighteenth century and others relating its unfolding starting in the second decade of the nineteenth century.
The concept was most fully elaborated by Charles Seller, *The Market Revolution: Jacksonian America, 1815–1846* (New York: Oxford University Press,
1990), as a synthesis of changes that reshaped American life during the
first half of the nineteenth century.

19. Master craftsmen became less involved in actual production, spending
more time on procuring materials and finding outlets for their goods.

20. I use the term "living wage" in preference to the term "family wage,"
which many historians have used. Lawrence B. Glickman points out that
workers themselves almost exclusively used "living wage" rather than
"family wage." Lawrence B. Glickman, *A Living Wage: American Workers
and the Making of Consumer Society* (Ithaca, NY: Cornell University Press,
1999), 158.

21. Joshua R. Greenberg, *Advocating the Man: Masculinity, Organized Labor, and
the Household in New York, 1800–1840* (New York: Columbia University
Press, 2008).

22. Martha May, "Bread before Roses: American Workingmen, Labor Unions
and the Family Wage," in Ruth Milkman, ed., *Women, Work and Protest:
A Century of U.S. Women's Labor History* (Boston: Routledge and Kegan
Paul, 1983), 4; Jean Boydston, "To Earn Her Daily Bread: Housework and
Antebellum Working-Class Subsistence," *Radical History Review* 35 (April
1986): 14.

23. Nancy Folbre, "The Unproductive Housewife: Her Evolution in Nineteenth
Century Economic Thought," *Signs* 16, no. 3 (1991): 466.

24. Boydston, "To Earn Her Daily Bread," 7–25.

25. Kessler-Harris, *Out to Work,* 56, 57.

26. Joel Perlman and Robert A. Margo, *Women's Work? American Schoolteachers,
1650–1920* (Chicago: University of Chicago Press, 2001), 55; Jo Anne Pres-
ton, "Domestic Ideology, School Reformers, and Female Teachers: School-
teaching Becomes Women's Work in Nineteenth-Century New England,"
The New England Quarterly 66, no. 4 (December 1993): 531–532.

27. Emily Abel, *Hearts of Wisdom: American Women Caring for Kin, 1850–1940*
(Cambridge, MA: Harvard University Press, 2002), 37–67.

28. "The Industrial Revolution," lecture by Katherine Osburn, Associate Professor of History, Tennessee Tech University, available at http://iweb.tntech.edu/kosburn/history-201/industrialization.htm (accessed July 19, 2009).

29. On the trend toward apprentices living separate from their masters see Bruce Laurie, *Artisans into Workers: Labor in Nineteenth Century America* (Urbana: University of Illinois Press, 1997), 35. Sean Wilentz, *Chants Democratic: New York City and the Rise of the American Working Class, 1788–1850* (New York: Oxford University Press, 1986), 48, notes that, by 1815, only 1 in 10 journeymen boarded with their masters.

30. Gunderson, *To Be Useful to the World,* 171 (speaking of women in the early republic, i.e., 1780s and 1790s).

31. Jeanne Boydston, *Home and Hearth: Housework, Wages and the Ideology of Labor in the Early Republic* (New York: Oxford University Press, 1990), 51–52.

32. Paul A. Gilje, "The Rise of Capitalism in the Early Republic," *Journal of the Early Republic* 16 (Summer 1996): 165–166. According to Gilje, a boom in turnpike building in the 1790s and early 1800s was followed by booms in canal building in the 1820s and 1830s and railroad construction in the 1840s and 1850s.

33. Alfred D. Chandler Jr. "The Emergence of Managerial Capitalism," *Business History Review* 58 (Winter 1984): 492–495.

34. Glickman, *A Living Wage,* 14.

35. Chandler, "The Emergence of Managerial Capitalism," 473.

36. Deborah M. Figart, Ellen Mutari, and Marilyn Power, "Breadwinners and Other Workers: Gender and Race-Ethnicity in the Evolution of the Labor Force," in Ellen Mutari and Deborah M. Figart, eds., *Women and the Economy* (Armonk, NY: M. E. Sharpe, 1999), 46, 47.

37. Fraser and Gordon, "A Genealogy of Dependence," 318.

38. Folbre, "The Unproductive Housewife," 464.

39. Christine Bose, *Women in 1900: Gateway to the Political Economy of the Twentieth Century* (Philadelphia: Temple University Press, 2001), 29–31.

40. Kessler-Harris, *Out to Work,* 110.

41. They did, however, support protective legislation setting minimum wages and maximum hours for women on the assumption that women lacked the wherewithal to bargain for themselves. Feminist historians have argued that the impact of protective legislation, whether intentional or not, was to reduce women's employment opportunities.

42. Eugene Debs, "The Common Laborer," *Terre Haute Locomotive Firemen's Magazine* 14, no. 4 (April 1890): 294, available at http://www.marxists.org/history/usa/unions/blf/1890/0400-debs-commonlaborer.pdf (accessed May 23, 2008).

43. David Montgomery, *The Fall of the House of Labor: The Workplace, the State, and American Labor Activism, 1865–1925* (Cambridge: Cambridge University Press, 1987), 60.

44. Ibid., 65.

45. U.S. Commissioner of Labor, *Sixth Annual Reports: Cost of Production* (Washington, DC: Government Printing Office, 1891), 693.

46. Robert W. Smuts, *Women and Work in America* (New York: Columbia University Press, 1959), 11; Tamara Hareven, *Amoskeag: Life and Work in an American Factory-City* (New York: Pantheon, 1978; reprint, Hanover, NH: University Press of New England, 1995), esp. 254–273.

47. Eileen Boris, *Home to Work: Motherhood and the Politics of Industrial Homework in the United States* (Cambridge: Cambridge University Press, 1994).

48. Laurence Glasco, "The Life Cycles and Household Structures of American Ethnic Groups: Irish, Germans, and Native-Born Whites in Buffalo, New York, 1855," in Nancy F. Cott and Elizabeth H. Pleck, eds., *A Heritage of Her Own: Toward a New Social History of American Women* (New York: Simon and Schuster, 1979), 268–289.

49. Elizabeth H. Pleck, "A Mother's Wages: Income Earning among Married Italian and Black Women, 1896–1911," in Nancy F. Cott and Elizabeth H. Pleck, eds., *A Heritage of Her Own: Toward a New Social History of American Women* (New York: Simon and Schuster, 1979), 367–392.

50. S. J. Kleinberg, "Children's and Mothers' Wage Labor in Three Eastern Cities, 1880–1920," *Social Science History* 29, no. 1 (Spring 2005): 69. Nonetheless, Kleinberg's findings also show that many African American families did not have the luxury of being able to do without children's earnings; thus African American children had the highest rates of labor force participation of all children (p. 54).

51. Ruth Schwartz Cowan, *More Work for Mother: The Ironies of Household Technology from the Open Hearth to the Microwave* (New York: Basic Books, 1983); Susan Strasser, *Never Done: A History of American Housework* (New York: Henry Holt, 1982), 104–125; Abel, *Hearts of Wisdom*, 46–48.

52. David Katzman, *Seven Days a Week: Women and Domestic Service in Industrial America* (New York: Oxford University Press, 1978), 286.

53. Aaron S. Fogleman, "From Slaves, Convicts, and Servants to Free Passengers: The Transformation of Immigration in the Era of the American Revolution," *The Journal of American History* (June 1998): 43.

54. Ira Berlin, *Many Thousands Gone: The First Two Centuries of Slavery in North America,* new ed. (Cambridge, MA: Belknap Press, 2000).

55. On the evolution of the legal status of blacks, especially black slaves in Virginia, see Leon Higginbotham, *In the Matter of Color: Race and the*

American Legal Process, The Colonial Period (New York: Oxford University Press, 1980), 19–58.

56. Native American slaves worked alongside white indentured servants and African slaves during the seventeenth and eighteenth centuries in South Carolina, and there was a flourishing Native American slave trade between the British Carolina region and the British Caribbean. The trade in Native American slaves declined in the early 1700s and ended by the 1750s because slave owners preferred Africans. However, Native Americans intermixed with African slaves, and many of their descendents went on to become slaves or slaveholders. See Alan Gallay, *The Indian Slave Trade: The Rise and Fall of the English Empire in the American South, 1670–1717* (New Haven, CT: Yale University Press, 2003); Tiya Miles, *Ties That Bind: The Story of an Afro-Cherokee Family in Slavery and Freedom* (Berkeley: University of California Press, 2005).

57. Berlin, *Many Thousands Gone,* 264–265, 308–309; Kenneth M. Stampp, *The Peculiar Institution: Slavery in the Ante-bellum South* (New York: Vintage, 1988), 32n.

58. Herbert S. Klein, *The Atlantic Slave Trade: A Census* (Cambridge: Cambridge University Press, 1999), 194; Robert William Fogel and Stanley L. Engerman, *Time on the Cross: The Economics of American Negro Slavery* (Boston: Little, Brown and Company, 1974), 76.

59. Jacqueline Jones, *Labor of Love, Labor of Sorrow: Black Women, Work, and Family from Slavery to the Present* (New York: Basic Books, 1985), 15–17, 19–20, 23; Deborah Gray White, *Ar'n't I a Woman: Female Slaves in the Plantation South,* 2nd ed. (New York: W. W. Norton, 1985), 115–117; Abel, *Hearts of Wisdom,* 62–63.

60. Vermont outlawed slavery in its constitution in 1777; language in the Massachusetts 1780 Constitution declaring all men being born equal and independent was interpreted by the courts as prohibiting slavery; New Hampshire's Constitution of 1783 contained language similar to the Massachusetts Constitution. However, there are no records indicating that New Hampshire courts construed the phrase as ending slavery, and slaves were still counted in the 1790 and 1800 censuses, albeit only eight in the latter. David Menschel, "Abolition without Deliverance: The Law of Connecticut Slavery 1784–1848," *The Yale Law Journal* 111, no. 1 (October 2001): 183; Joanne Pope Melish, *Disowning Slavery: Gradual Emancipation and Race in New England, 1780–1860* (Ithaca, NY: Cornell University Press, 1998).

61. The respective dates were Pennsylvania (1780), Connecticut (1784), Rhode Island (1784), New York (1799), and New Jersey (1804). Menschel, "Abolition without Deliverance," 183, 188. See also David Nathaniel Gellman,

Emancipating New York (Baton Rouge: Louisiana State University Press, 2006), 176–183.

62. Menschel, "Abolition without Deliverance," Connecticut (1848) and New Jersey (1846). For a review of individual states and comparative information on abolition of slavery by northern states, see "Slavery in the North," http://www.slavenorth.com/ (accessed July 8, 2009).

63. Hartigan-O'Connor, "'She Said She Did Not Know Money,'" 332.

64. Fogleman, "From Slaves, Convicts, and Servants to Free Passengers," 44, 45; Kenneth Morgan, *Slavery and Servitude in Colonial North America, A Short History* (New York: New York University Press, 2000), 45–47.

65. Fogleman, "From Slaves, Convicts, and Servants to Free Passengers," 44, 46, 47.

66. For example, according to Sharon Salinger the proportion of female indentured servants in Philadelphia rose from less than 20 percent in the mid-eighteenth century to 30 percent shortly before the Revolution and to nearly 40 percent by 1795: Sharon V. Salinger, *"To Serve Well and Faithfully": Labor and Indentured Servants in Philadelphia* (Cambridge: Cambridge University Press, 1987), 138–139.

67. Ibid., 100.

68. Ibid., 150–151.

69. Ibid., 129.

70. A. Roger Ekirch, *Bound for America: The Transportation of British Convicts to the Colonies, 1718–1775* (Oxford: Oxford University Press, 1987); Farley Grubb, "The Transatlantic Market for British Convict Labor," *Journal of Economic History* 60, no. 1 (March 2000): 94–122; Morgan, *Slavery and Servitude in Colonial North America,* 48–49.

71. David W. Galenson, "The Rise and Fall of Indentured Servitude in the Americas: An Economic Analysis," *The Journal of Economic History,* 44, no. 1 (March 1984): 13.

72. Ian M. G. Quimby, *Apprenticeship in Colonial Philadelphia* (New York: Garland, 1985), 99–126; John E. Murray and Ruth Wallis Herndon, "Markets for Children in Early America: A Political Economy of Pauper Apprenticeship," *The Journal of Economic History* 62, no. 2 (June 2002): 356–382.

73. Karin L. Zipf, *Labor of Innocents: Forced Apprenticeship in North Carolina, 1715–1919* (Baton Rouge: Louisiana State University Press, 2005), 12–16; Murray and Herndon, "Markets for Children in Early America," 356–361.

74. Fogleman, "From Slaves, Convicts, and Servants to Free Passengers," 62–63; Salinger, *"To Serve Well and Faithfully,"* 151–152.

75. Gordon S. Wood, *Radicalism of the American Revolution* (New York: Vintage, 1993), 145, 184; Robert J. Steinfeld, *The Invention of Free Labor: The*

Employment Relation in English and American Law and Culture, 1350–1870 (Chapel Hill: University of North Carolina Press, 1991).

76. Eric Foner, *Reconstruction: America's Unfinished Revolution, 1863–1877* (New York: Harper & Row, 1988), 176–298; William Cohen, *At Freedom's Edge: Black Mobility and the Southern White Quest for Racial Control* (Baton Rouge: Louisiana State University Press, 1991), 53; W. E. B. Du Bois, *Black Reconstruction in America* (New York: Oxford University Press, 2007), 611.

77. Michael Perman, *Struggle for Mastery: Disfranchisement in the South, 1888–1908* (Chapel Hill: University of North Carolina Press, 2001), 10–17, 15; Leon F. Litwack, *Trouble in Mind: Black Southerners in the Age of Jim Crow* (New York: Knopf, 1998), 284–298, 312–319, 406–410.

78. Cohen, *At Freedom's Edge,* 16, 20–21; Jones, *Labor of Love,* 58–61; Foner, *Reconstruction,* 173–174; Roger L. Ransom and Richard Sutch, *One Kind of Freedom: The Economic Consequences of Emancipation* (Cambridge: Cambridge University Press, 1977), 87–88, 68–70.

79. Robert B. Outland, *Tapping the Pines: The Naval Stores Industry in the American South* (Baton Rouge: Louisiana State University Press, 2004), 162–173.

80. Tera W. Hunter, "Domination and Resistance: The Politics of Wage Household Labor in New South Atlanta," *Labor History* 34 (Spring/Summer 1993): 257–258; Walter F. White, "'Work or Fight' in the South," in Herbert Aptheker, ed., *A Documentary History of the Negro People in the United States,* vol. 3 (New York: Citadel Press, 1993), 238–239.

81. John Dittmer, *Black Georgia in the Progressive Era, 1900–1920* (Urbana: University of Illinois Press, 1977), 76–77; Pete Daniels, *The Shadow of Slavery: Peonage in the South, 1901–1969* (Urbana: University of Illinois Press, 1972), 23–29; William C. Cohen, "Negro Involuntary Servitude in the South, 1865–1940: A Preliminary Analysis," *Journal of Southern History* 42, no. 1 (February 1976): 47–51; Jacqueline Jones, *American Work: Four Centuries of Black and White Labor* (New York: Norton, 1998), 316–317.

82. St. Clair Drake and Horace Cayton, *Black Metropolis: A Study of Negro Life in a Northern City,* rev. ed. (Chicago: University of Chicago Press, 1993), 214–262.

83. Unlike other black service workers, Pullman porters were unionized and relatively well paid, and thus were especially esteemed in the black community. See Jack Santino, *Miles of Smiles, Years of Struggle: Stories of Black Pullman Porters* (Urbana: University of Illinois Press, 1989), 7–8, 12–17; Beth Tompkin Bates, *Pullman Porters and the Rise of Protest Politics in Black America, 1925–1945* (Chapel Hill: University of North Carolina Press, 2001), 10; Edward Berman, "The Pullman Porters Win," *Nation* 141 (August 21, 1935), 217.

84. Jones, *Labor of Love, Labor of Sorrow,* 160–182.

85. Sarah Deutsch, *No Separate Refuge: Culture, Class, and Gender on an Anglo-Hispanic Frontier in the American Southwest, 1880–1940* (New York: Oxford University Press, 1987), 22–23.

86. Neil Foley, *The White Scourge: Mexicans, Blacks, and Poor Whites in Texas Cotton Culture* (Berkeley: University of California Press, 1997), 127.

87. Deutsch, *No Separate Refuge,* 91.

88. Mark Reisler, *By the Sweat of Their Brow: Mexican Labor in the United States, 1900–1940* (Westport, CT: Greenwood Press, 1976), 10, 82.

89. Paul M. Ong, "The Central Pacific Railroad and Exploitation of Chinese Labor," *Journal of Ethnic Studies* 13, no. 2 (1985): 119–124; Alexander Saxton, "The Army of Canton in the High Sierra," *Pacific Historical Review* 35, no. 2 (1966): 141–151. On the credit ticket system see Gunther Peck, *Reinventing Free Labor: Padrones and Immigrant Workers in North America* (Cambridge: Cambridge University Press, 2000), 51–52.

90. Robert J. Steinfeld, *Coercion, Contract, and Free Labor in the Nineteenth Century* (Cambridge: Cambridge University Press, 2001), 307–308.

91. Ibid., 312. Steinfeld argues against the common belief that wage labor was equivalent to free labor. Moreover, he throws into question any natural difference between free and unfree labor, arguing that the line between them has been drawn differently in different countries and different historical periods.

92. Abel, *Hearts of Wisdom,* 40, 39, 52, 38.

93. Ibid., 43, 45.

94. Wilma A. Dunaway, *The African American Family in Slavery and Emancipation* (New York: Cambridge University Press, 2003), 152, 153.

95. Abel, *Hearts of Wisdom,* 61, 63, 64, 65. The slave narrator was quite correct: calomel is mercury chloride, commonly used as a purgative or insecticide in the nineteenth century. It is highly toxic.

96. Paul Starr, *The Social Transformation of American Medicine: The Rise of a Sovereign Profession and the Making of a Vast Industry,* (New York: Basic Books, 1982), 102–127, 108–110, 120. According to Starr, the medical profession became more homogeneous—i.e., white Christian male—since women's medical schools and black medical schools were disproportionately among the "marginal" schools that closed down, and the remaining schools systematically discriminated against Jews, blacks, and women (ibid., 124).

97. Susan Reverby, *Ordered to Care: The Dilemma of American Nursing, 1850–1945* (New York: Cambridge University Press, 1985), 61, 121–142; Starr, *Social Transformation of American Medicine,* 119–120.

98. Abel, *Hearts of Wisdom,* 121, 122, 126–148.

3. The Movement to Reform Women's Caring

1. Nicole Hahn Rafter, *Partial Justice: Women in State Prisons, 1800–1935* (Boston: Northeastern University Press, 1985), 53.

2. See John Whiteclay Chambers II, *The Tyranny of Change: America in the Progressive Era,* 2nd ed. (New Brunswick, NJ: Rutgers University Press, 2000), chapter 5.

3. See Peggy Pascoe, *Relations of Rescue: The Search for Female Moral Authority in the American West, 1874–1939* (New York: Oxford University Press, 1990); Estelle Friedman, *Their Sisters' Keepers: Women's Prison Reform in America, 1830–1930* (Ann Arbor: University of Michigan Press, 1981); Barbara Epstein, *The Politics of Domesticity: Women, Evangelism, and Temperance in Nineteenth-Century America* (Middletown, CT: Wesleyan University Press, 1981); Ruth Rosen, *The Lost Sisterhood: Prostitution in America, 1900–1918* (Baltimore, MD: Johns Hopkins University Press, 1982); Evelyn Brooks Higginbotham, *Righteous Discontent: The Women's Movement in the Black Baptist Church, 1880–1920* (Cambridge, MA: Harvard University Press, 1994); Ellen Fitzpatrick, *Endless Crusade: Women Social Scientists and Progressive Reform* (New York: Oxford University Press, 1994); Robyn Munch, *Creating a Female Dominion in American Reform, 1890–1935* (New York: Oxford University Press, 1994).

4. The commonly used term in the early twentieth century was "Americanization," a particularly ironic designation for people who are now called "Native Americans." However, because the term "Americanization" has been more commonly used to refer to programs designed to acculturate immigrants, I use the term "assimilation" in this chapter to refer to policies and programs designed to "deculturalize" Native Americans and force-fit them into subordinate positions in American society. The ultimate aim was to disempower them as nations and as peoples by terminating collective landholding and tribal rights.

5. See Frederick E. Hoxie, *A Final Promise: The Campaign to Assimilate the Indians, 1880–1920* (Lincoln: University of Nebraska Press, 2001) for an overview. See also Kenneth H. Bobroff, "Retelling Allotment: Indian Property Rights and the Myth of Common Ownership," *Vanderbilt Law Review* 54, no. 4 (2001): 1567.

6. Carl Schurz, Secretary of the Interior under Rutherford B. Hayes, expressed these ideas in an article, "Aspects of the Indian Problem," in the *North American Review* in 1881, excerpted in Francis Paul Prucha, ed., *Americanizing the American Indians* (Cambridge, MA: Harvard University Press, 1973), 13–26, esp. 20.

7. Allison M. Dussias, "Squaw Drudges, Farm Wives, and the Dann Sisters' Last Stand: American Indian Women's Resistance to Domestication and

the Denial of Their Property Rights," *North Carolina Law Review* 77 (January 1999): 676.

8. Rose Stremlau, "'To Domesticate and Civilize Wild Indians': Allotment and the Campaign to Reform Indian Families, 1875–1887," *Journal of Family History* 30, no. 3 (July 2005): 271–273; *Annual Report of the Commissioner of Indian Affairs (1893)* (Washington, DC: Government Printing Office, 1893), 55.

9. Mrs. Merial A. Dorchester, "Suggestions from the Field to the Honorable Superintendent of Indian Schools," in *Annual Report of the Commissioner of Indian Affairs (1891)* (Washington, DC: Government Printing Office, 1891), 542.

10. Margaret D. Jacobs, *Engendered Encounters: Feminism and Pueblo Cultures, 1879–1934* (Lincoln: University of Nebraska Press, 1999), 24–55.

11. David D. Smits, "The 'Squaw Drudge': A Prime Index of Savagism," *Ethnohistory* 29, no. 4 (1982): 281–306, esp. 298–300. In the latter half of the nineteenth century the emerging social sciences reinforced the presumed inferiority of indigenous societies by hierarchically ranking societies along an evolutionary scale from the most primitive to the most advanced. In his influential book, *Ancient Society,* Anthropologist Lewis Henry Morgan identified three stages of societal evolution, savagery, barbarism, and civilization, correlating each stage with a particular family form. According to Morgan, the monogamous patrilineal family, which characterized European and North American societies, was the mark of civilization, having emerged only when it became necessary to assure paternity and regularize the inheritance of property. In his opinion, the most progressive American Indians were at no higher stage than that of middle barbarism. See Lewis Henry Morgan, *Ancient Society,* ed. Eleanor B. Leacock (1877; reprint, Cleveland: World Publishing Company, 1963), 67.

12. *1888 Report of the Commissioner of Indian Affairs* (Washington, DC: Government Printing Office, 1889), lxxix; Dussias, "Squaw Drudges, Farm Wives," 697; Jacobs, *Engendered Encounters,* 34.

13. Catherine Haun, "A Woman's Trip across the Plains in 1849," in Lillian Schlissel, ed., *Women's Diaries of the Westward Journey* (New York: Schocken Books, 1992), 174–175; Margaret D. Jacobs, "Maternal Colonialism: White Women and Indigenous Child Removal in the American West and Australia, 1880–1940," *The Western Historical Quarterly* 36 (Winter 2005): 463–464.

14. *1893 Report of the Commissioner of Indian Affairs* (Washington, DC: Government Printing Office, 1894), 55.

15. Dussias, "Squaw Drudges, Farm Wives," 674, notes that the particular reservations were selected for the allotment program in response to pressure from whites for access to lands in specific areas.

16. D. S. Otis, *The Dawes Act and the Allotment of Indian Lands,* ed. Francis Paul Prucha (Cambridge, MA: Harvard University Press, 1973), 10–11.

17. Report of the Superintendent of Indian Schools, in *Annual Report of the Commissioner of Indian Affairs (1900)* (Washington, DC: Government Printing Office, 1900), 426, 427.

18. Descriptions of programs for domestic training for girls, along with commentary about the purpose of such training, appear in the reports of the superintendents of the various Indian schools that are included in the *Annual Reports of the Commissioner of Indian Affairs.* For example, the superintendent of the Oneida school, in his 1900 report, noted: "The girls receive the usual training in sewing, cooking, washing, and housework, and I doubt if there is any more lasting benefit that can be conferred upon them than giving them instruction in the old-fashioned but very necessary home duties. A clean house and well-cooked meals are very attractive to men, and who can say but what the influence of a pretty home and dainty table may go far toward overcoming the temptation to drink and evil associations that have so long hindered progress here as elsewhere?" (ibid., 513).

19. Margaret D. Jacobs, *White Mother to a Dark Race: Settler Colonialism, Maternalism and Removal of Indigenous Children in the American West and Australia, 1880–1940* (Lincoln: University of Nebraska Press, 2005), 136.

20. Jacobs, "Maternal Colonialism," 59; Joan T. Mark, *A Stranger in Her Native Land: Alice Fletcher and the American Indians* (Lincoln: University of Nebraska Press, 1989), 79.

21. Robert A. Trennert, "Educating Indian Girls at Nonreservation Boarding Schools, 1878–1920," *The Western Historical Quarterly* 13, no. 3 (July 1982): 273–274.

22. Ibid., 274, 275.

23. Ibid., 275; *Annual Report of the Commissioner of Indian Affairs (1880)* (Washington, DC: Government Printing Office, 1880), 180, 182–183; R. H. Pratt, *The Indian Industrial School, Carlisle, Pennsylvania: Its Origins, Purposes, Progress, and the Difficulties Surmounted,* reprint of 1908 text (Carlisle, PA: Cumberland Historical Society, 1979), 28.

24. Trennert, "Educating Indian Girls," 275; *Annual Report of the Commissioner of Indian Affairs (1881)* (Washington, DC: Government Printing Office, 1881), 188–189.

25. John Reyhmer and Jeanne Eder, *American Indian Education: A History* (Norman: University of Oklahoma Press, 2004), tables 1 and 2, 150–151; Trennert, "Educating Indian Girls," 283.

26. Reyhmer and Eder, *American Indian Education,* tables 1 and 2, 150–151.

27. *Annual Report of the Commissioner of Indian Affairs (1889)* (Washington, DC: Government Printing Office, 1889), 93–114; *Annual Report of the*

Commissioner of Indian Affairs (1890) (Washington, DC: Government Printing Office, 1890), cxlvi–clvi.

28. Trennert, "Educating Indian Girls," 281.
29. Estelle Reel, *Course of Study for the Indian Schools, Industrial and Literary* (Washington, DC: Government Printing Office, 1901); K. Tsianina Lomawaima, "Domesticity in the Federal Indian Schools: The Power of Authority over Mind and Body," *American Ethnologist* 20, no. 1 (February 1993); Trennert, "Educating Indian Girls," 282.
30. David Wallace Adams, *Education for Extinction: American Indians and the Boarding School Experience, 1875–1928* (Lawrence: University Press of Kansas, 1995), 149–156.
31. Reel, *Course of Study,* 189; Robert A. Trennert, "From Carlisle to Phoenix: The Rise and Fall of the Indian Outing System, 1878–1930," *Pacific Historical Review* 52, no. 3 (August 1983): 267–291; Trennert, "Educating Indian Girls," 283; "Report of School at Carlisle PA," in *Annual Report of the Commissioner of Indian Affairs (1900),* 509. See Adams, *Education for Extinction,* 156–163, and Brenda J. Childs, *Boarding School Seasons: American Indian Families, 1900–1940* (Lincoln: University of Nebraska Press, 1998), 81–86, for Indian students' perspectives on the outing system.
32. W. Roger Buffalohead and Paulette Fairbanks Molin, "'A Nucleus of Civilization': American Indian Families at Hampton Institute in the Late Nineteenth Century," *Journal of American Indian Education* 35, no. 3 (May 1996): 59–94; Josephine E. Richards, "The Training of the Indian Girl as the Uplifter of the Home," *Journal of Proceedings and Addresses of the Thirty-Ninth Annual Meeting* (National Educational Association, 1900), 701–705. See K. Tsianina Lomawaima, "Estelle Reel, Superintendent of Indian Schools, 1898–1910," *Journal of American Indian Education* 35, no. 3 (May 1996): 14–15, for Indian women's memories of the industrial or "practice" cottage system. The cost of erecting the cottages had been raised by the Connecticut Indian Women's Association. The Association went on to develop a loan program to lend money to Indian couples who had attended Hampton to build Western style houses on their allotment land (Buffalohead and Molin, "'A Nucleus of Civilization,'" 62, 75–79).
33. Richards, *The Training of Indian Girls,* 702–703; K. Tsianina Lomawaima, *They Called It Prairie Light: The Story of Chilocco Indian School* (Lincoln: University of Nebraska Press, 1994), 88.
34. Adams, "Schooling the Hopi: Federal Indian Policy Writ Small, 1887–1917," *Pacific Historical Reveiew* 48, no. 3 (August 1979): 340–342.
35. Ibid., 335–356; Childs, *Boarding School Seasons,* 90–91.
36. Jacobs, "White Mother," 15.
37. Adams, *Education for Extinction,* 130–133.

38. Ibid., 224–228, 229–231; Childs, *Boarding School Seasons,* 93.

39. Adams, *Education for Extinction,* 233–234.

40. For example, Michael C. Coleman, *American Indian Children at School, 1850–1930* (Jackson: University of Mississippi Press, 2007), based on more than 50 memoirs and autobiographies.

41. Adams, *Education for Extinction,* 153.

42. Ibid., 184, 187.

43. Child, *Boarding School Seasons,* xiv, 3–4, 76.

44. *Proceedings of the 11th Annual Meeting of the Lake Mohonk Conference of the Friends of the Indian (1893)* (n.p.: Lake Mohonk Conference, 1893), 30.

45. Jacobs, *White Mother to a Dark Race,* 403–404.

46. Trennert, "Educating Indian Girls," 286–288.

47. Sally Hyer, *One House, One Voice, One Heart: Native American Education at the Santa Fe Indian School* (Santa Fe: The Museum of New Mexico, 1990).

48. Estelle B. Freedman, *Their Sisters' Keepers: Women's Prison Reform in America, 1830–1930* (Ann Arbor: University of Michigan Press, 1981), 11; L. Mara Dodge, "'One Female Prisoner Is of More Trouble than Twenty Males': Women Convicts in Illinois Prisons, 1835–1896," *Journal of Social History* 32, no. 4 (Summer 1999): 907.

49. Nicole Hahn Rafter, "Prisons for Women, 1790–1980," in Michael Tonry and Norval Morris, eds., *Crime and Justice: An Annual Review of Research,* vol. 5 (Chicago: The University of Chicago Press, 1983), 136–140.

50. Freedman, *Their Sisters' Keepers,* 11.

51. Ibid., 12–13, 16.

52. Larry Whiteaker, *Seduction, Prostitution, and Moral Reform in New York, 1830–1860* (New York: Routledge, 1997). On lady visitors to New York's Bellevue Prison, see 46–47.

53. Barbara M. Brenzel, *Daughters of the State: A Social Portrait of the First Reform School for Girls in North America, 1856–1905* (Cambridge, MA: MIT Press, 1983), 81, 119–122, 72–73.

54. Eugenia Cornelia Lekkerkerker, *Reformatories for Women in the United States* (Groningen: B. J. Wolters' Uitgevers-maatschappij, 1931), 91.

55. Isabel C. Barrows, "The Massachusetts Reformatory Prison for Women," in *The Reformatory System of the United States,* Report for the International Prison Commission (Washington, DC: Government Printing Office, 1900), 108.

56. Nicole Hahn Rafter, *Partial Justice: Women, Prisons, and Social Control* (New Brunswick, NJ: Transaction Publishers, 1990), 13, 49.

57. Rebecca Burkholder, "Massachusetts Reformatory for Women: The Superintendents, 1877–1930," unpublished paper (1988), 5–6, available by request

from Georgetown University School of Law at http://www.law.georgetown
.edu/glh/index.html#papers (accessed June 18, 2009).

58. Ibid., 5.

59. Rafter, *Partial Justice,* 25–26.

60. Barrows, "The Massachusetts Reformatory Prison for Women," 106.

61. Rafter, "Prisons for Women," 155; Rafter, *Partial Justice,* 56, table 3.1.

62. Rafter, *Partial Justice,* 36.

63. Nicole Hahn Rafter, "Gender, Prisons, and Prison History," *Social Science History* 9, no. 3 (Summer 1985): 240; Rafter, *Partial Justice,* 143, 150–152.

64. Freedman, *Their Sisters' Keepers,* 139.

65. Rafter, "Gender, Prisons, and Prison History," 139–141.

66. Freedman, *Their Sisters' Keepers,* 87.

67. Nicole Hahn Rafter, "Chastising the Unchaste: Social Control Functions of a Women's Reformatory, 1894–1931," in Stanley Cohen and Andrew Scull, eds., *Social Control and the State: Historical and Comparative Essays* (Oxford: Martin Robertson, 1983), 29; Rafter, *Partial Justice,* xviii.

68. Freedman, *Their Sisters' Keepers,* 131, 61, 68; Barrows, "The Massachusetts Reformatory," 120, quoting 1896 report by the superintendent.

69. Rafter, "Gender, Prisons, and Prison History," 236–237.

70. Rafter, *Partial Justice,* 33–34; Freedman, *Their Sisters' Keepers,* 131–132, 133.

71. Rafter, *Partial Justice,* 39.

72. Burkholder, "Massachusetts Reformatory for Women," 40.

73. Ellen C. Johnson, "Prison Discipline," in *The Reformatory System of the United States,* Report for the International Prison Commission (Washington, DC: Government Printing Office, 1900), 132–133.

74. Barrows, "The Massachusetts Reformatory," 120–121, quoting the 1896 report of the superintendent, Ellen Cheney Johnson.

75. Rafter, *Partial Justice,* 39–40.

76. Ibid., 38.

77. State v. Heitman, 105 Kan. 139, 146, 147. The court further noted in support of its position, "Since 1859 some thirteen other states have established separate institutions for the treatment of delinquent women on the definite principle of reclamation as opposed to naked punishment. The industrial farm, with buildings constructed on the cottage plan, has become an accepted type, and the indeterminate sentence has been almost, though not quite, universally adopted."

78. Freedman, *Their Sisters' Keepers,* 92, 93.

79. Ibid., 163–165.

80. Johnson, "Prison Discipline," 131, 132.

81. Barrows, "The Massachusetts Reformatory," 122, 123, 124.

82. Freedman, *Their Sisters' Keepers,* 149.

83. See ibid., 109–125, for an extended discussion of the new thinking.

84. Rafter, "Prisons for Women," 165.

85. John Higham, *Strangers in the Land: Patterns of American Nativism, 1860–1925* (New Brunswick, NJ: Rutgers University Press, 1963), 234; John F. McClymer, "The Americanization Movement and the Education of the Foreign-Born Adult, 1914–1925," in Bernard J. Weiss, ed., *American Education and the European Immigrant, 1840–1940* (Urbana: University of Illinois Press, 1982), 96–97.

86. Higham, *Strangers in the Land,* 236–237. See Robert A. Woods and Albert J. Kennedy, *Handbook of Settlements* (New York: Russell Sage Foundation, 1911), for descriptions of activities of 413 settlement houses based on a survey conducted by the Russell Sage Foundation.

87. Gayle Gullett, "Women Progressives and the Politics of Americanization in California, 1915–1920," *Pacific Historical Review* 64 (February 1995): 72, 80, 79.

88. Higham, *Strangers in the Land,* 236.

89. Ibid., 236–237, 247.

90. McClymer, "Gender and the American Way of Life"; Stephen Meyer, "Adapting the Immigrant to the Line: Americanization in the Ford Factory, 1914–1921," *Journal of Social History* 14, no. 1 (Fall 1980): 67–82; Clinton C. DeWitt, "Industrial Teachers," in United States Bureau of Education, *Proceedings, Americanization Conference* (Washington, DC: Government Printing Office, 1916), 119.

91. Seth Korelitz, "'A Magnificent Piece of Work': The Americanization Work of the National Council of Jewish Women," *American Jewish History* 83, no. 2 (June 1995): 177–203. On Ford, see Meyer, "Adapting the Immigrant to the Line: Americanization in the Ford Factory, 1914–1921," *Journal of Social History* 14, no. 1 (Fall 1980): 67–82. On B. F. Goodrich, see *National Association of Corporation Schools Bulletin (NACSB)* 6, no. 7 (July 1919): 322; *NACSB* 6, no. 10 (October 1919): 466–467; *NACSB* 7, no. 6 (June 1920): 276–277. On Westinghouse, see *NACSB* 7 no. 3 (March 1920): 105–107. On General Electric, see "Americanization Developments Are Getting Satisfactory Results," *NACSB* 7, no. 30 (March 1920): 109–113; *National Association of Corporation Training Bulletin (NACTB)* 8, no. 1 (January 1921): 44; *NACTB* 8, no. 2 (February 1921): 87; *NACTB* 8, no. 4 (April 1921): 182; *NACSB* 6, no. 10 (October 1919): 466; *NACSB* 7, no. 3 (March 1920): 105. See also McClymer, "The Americanization Movement," 98.

92. Gerd Korman, "Americanization at the Factory Gate," *Industrial and Labor Relations Review* 18, no. 3 (April 1965): 404–409; Higham, *Strangers in the Land,* 239, 258.

93. Gullett, "Women Progressives," 80–81.
94. McClymer, "Gender and the American Way of Life," 4; "List of Those Attending Americanization Conference" (May 12–15, 1919), in *Proceedings, Americanization Conference* (Washington, DC: Government Printing Office, 1919), 7–20.
95. McClymer, "Gender and the American Way of Life," 4–5.
96. Gullett, "Women Progressives," 75, 76.
97. Helen Varick Boswell, "Promoting Americanization," *Annals of the American Academy of Political and Social Science* 64 (March 1916): 206; McClymer, "Gender and the American Way of Life," 4.
98. Gullett, "Women Progressives," 73; Gertrude Van Hoesen, "The Relation of the Home-Economics Workers to the Problems of the Foreign Woman," in *Proceedings of the Americanization Conference,* comp. Americanization Division, U.S. Bureau of Education (Washington, DC: Government Printing Office, 1919), 406.
99. Frank V. Thompson, *Schooling of the Immigrant* (New York: Harper & Bros., 1920).
100. "The Home Teacher Act," in *The Home Teacher: The Act with a Working Plan and Forty Lessons in English,* Commission of Immigration and Housing of California (Sacramento, CA: California State Printing Office, 1916), 4.
101. At the end of the pamphlet there are brief reports from Americanization projects around the country. These reports confirm that local programs for the most part adhered to the suggested focus on household topics by offering sewing and cooking classes, English lessons, and social events and outings. Only one report, from Los Angeles, lists classes in citizenship along with those in sewing, cooking, and English. Bureau of Naturalization, U.S. Department of Labor, *Suggestions for Americanization Work among Foreign-Born Women* (Washington, DC: Government Printing Office, 1921), 6–8, 8–12.
102. Amanda Matthews Chase, *Primer for Foreign Speaking Women,* part I, Commission of Immigration and Housing of California (Sacramento: California State Printing Office, 1918), 10–32.
103. Pearl Idelia Ellis, *Americanization through Homemaking* (Los Angeles: Wetzel Publishing, 1929), 19, 26.
104. Boswell, "Promoting Americanization," 206; McClymer, "Gender and the American Way of Life," 12.
105. Ellis, *Americanization through Homemaking,* 29.
106. Annie L. Hansen, "Two Years as a Domestic Educator in Buffalo, New York," *Journal of Home Economics* (December 1913): 434, 435.
107. Grace A. Farrell, "Homemaking with the 'Other Half' along our International Border," *Journal of Home Economics* 21, no. 6 (June 1929): 413–414, 415.

108. Gullett, "Women Progressives," 85–86; Suellen Hoy, *Chasing Dirt: The American Pursuit of Cleanliness* (New York: Oxford University Press, 1995), 114; Lillian D. Wald, *The House on Henry Street* (New York: Henry Holt and Co., 1915), 108.

109. Mabel Hyde Kittredge, *Housekeeping Notes: How to Furnish and Keep House in a Tenement Flat* (Boston: Whitcomb & Barrows, 1911), 13.

110. Hoy, *Chasing Dirt,* 116–117.

111. Elizabeth Ewen, *Immigrant Women in the Land of Dollars: Life and Culture on the Lower East Side, 1890–1925* (New York: Monthly Review Press, 1985), 94; Gullett, "Women Progressives," 81–82.

112. Kittredge, *Housekeeping Notes,* 44–45. See also Ellis, *Americanization through Homemaking,* 33.

113. George J. Sanchez, " 'Go after the Women': Americanization and the Mexican American Woman, 1915–1929," in Vicki L. Ruiz and Ellen Carol DuBois, eds., *Unequal Sisters: A Multicultural Reader in U.S. Women's History,* 2nd ed. (New York: Routledge, 1994), 289.

114. Chase, *Primer for Foreign Speaking Women,* 33.

115. Maxine Seller, "Education of the Immigrant Woman: 1900–1935," *Journal of Urban History* 4 (1978): 317; Gullett, "Women Progressives," 90.

116. Higham, *Strangers in the Land,* 253–254, 300–301; David George Herman, *Neighbors on Gold Mountain: The Americanization of Immigrants in California* (PhD diss., University of California, Berkeley, 1981), 7.

117. Higham, *Strangers in the Land,* 324.

118. Spain gave up Cuba, granting it independence, ceded Puerto Rico and Guam to the United States, and "sold" the Philippines to the United States for $20 million.

119. William McKinley, *State of the Union Address,* December 3, 1900, part II, p. 4, http://teachingamericanhistory.org/library/index.asp?/documentpring=1205.

120. K. Tsianina Lomawaima, "Estelle Reel, Superintendent of Indian Schools, 1898–1910: Politics, Curriculum, and Land," *Journal of American Indian Education* 35, no. 3 (May 1996): 12.

121. Sonia M. Rosa, "The Puerto Ricans at Carlisle Indian School," in Lourdes Diaz Soto, ed., *The Praeger Handbook of Latino Education in the United States* (Westport, CT: Praeger, 2006), 386–391.

122. Elsie Mae Willsey, "Home Economics in Porto Rico," *Journal of Home Economics* 14, no. 11 (November 1922): 529.

123. Elvess Ann Sewart, "Home Economics in the Philippine Islands," *Journal of Home Economics* 21, no. 4 (April 1929): 237, 238, 242.

124. Agnes Hunt, "Domestic Science in Hawaii," *Journal of Home Economics* (September 1936): 642. I am grateful to Randall Roth for pointing me to materials on vocational education at the Kamehameha School.

125. Loring Hudson, "Homemaking in a Hawaiian School," *Journal of Home Economics* 28 (September 1936): 451; J. Arthur Rath, *Lost Generations: A Boy, A School, A Princess* (Honolulu: University of Hawai'i Press, 2005), 118. Interestingly, in the 1980s, 1990s, and 2000s the Kamehameha School in Honolulu became a key site for a strong assertion of traditional Native Hawaiian culture, for militancy on issues of Native Hawaiian sovereignty, and for incorporation of traditional Hawaiian culture into a highly competitive K–12 curriculum. The Kamehameha Schools have also established major new campuses on the islands of Hawai'i and Maui so as to better serve Native Hawaiian communities in those areas.

126. Darlene Clark Hine, "'We Specialize in the Wholly Impossible': The Philanthropic Work of Black Women," in Kathleen D. McCarthy, ed., *Lady Bountiful Revisited: Women, Philanthropy and Power* (New Brunswick, NJ: Rutgers University Press, 1990), 76.

127. Ibid., 75.

128. Ibid., 88.

129. Gayle Ann Gullett, *Becoming Citizens: The Emergence and Development of the California Women's Movement, 1880–1911* (Urbana: University of Illinois Press, 2000), 3–12, 19.

4. From Moral Duty to Legal Obligation

1. This is not to deny that men get involved in caring but to point out that they do so mostly as helpers rather than as the person mainly responsible for initiating care.

2. Emily K. Abel, *Who Cares for the Elderly? Public Policy and the Experiences of Adult Daughters* (Philadelphia: Temple University Press, 1991), 91; Karen V. Hansen, "The Asking Rules of Reciprocity in Networks of Care for Children," *Qualitative Sociology* 27, no. 4 (Winter 2004): 434; Jane Aronson, "Women's Sense of Responsibility for the Care of Old People: 'But Who Else Is Going to Do It?'" *Gender and Society* 6, no. 1 (March 1992): 15; Judith Globerman, "Motivations to Care: Daughters- and Sons-in-Law Caring for Relatives with Alzheimer's Disease," *Family Relations* 45, no. 1 (January 1996): 41.

3. Clare Ungerson, *Policy Is Personal: Sex, Gender, and Informal Care* (London: Tavistock Publications, 1987), 89; Isabela Paoletti, "Membership Categories and Time Appraisal in Interviews with Family Caregivers of Disabled Elderly," *Human Subjects* 24 (2001): 298.

4. Ungerson, *Policy Is Personal*, 51.

5. Isabel Paoletti, "Caring for Older People: A Gendered Practice," *Discourse and Society* 13 (2002): 813; Aronson, "Women's Sense of Responsibility for the Care of Old People," 19.

6. Globerman, "Motivations to Care," 41.

7. *Blackstone's Commentaries on the Laws of England,* Book the First—Chapter the Fifteenth: Of Husband and Wife, 430, The Avalon Project at Yale Law School, available at http://www.yale.edu/lawweb/avalon/blackstone/bk1ch15 .htm (accessed February 11, 2007).

8. A Delaware Superior Court decision of 1886, for example, spelled out the duties in this way: "It was her duty, as a wife, to do and superintend the doings of all such acts and things as were necessary for the due and proper management of the domestic concerns of the household, so far as her ability enabled her, and the means supplied her by her husband were adequate for the purpose. This includes among other things the keeping of the house in good and clean condition, the proper cooking and furnishing at reasonable hours of food for her husband and the children of the household, due attention to their wardrobe, and nursing and attention to them in sickness." Hogg v. Lobb's Executor, 32 A. 631 (Superior Court of Delaware, 1886), 400.

9. Under the doctrine of necessaries, "The husband is bound to provide his wife with necessaries by law, as much as himself; and if he contracts debts for them, he is obliged to pay them." (*Blackstone's Commentaries,* Book the First—Chapter the Fifteenth: Of Husband and Wife, 430). Thus a wife was entitled to obtain necessaries from a third party and charge them in her husband's name. The doctrine of necessaries was intended to enforce the support obligation on husbands who had the means to fulfill this duty but refused to do so. This mechanism was a thin reed on which to hang a woman's right to support because it required that third parties would agree to provide goods knowing that they might have great difficulty collecting from a recalcitrant spouse. ("The Unnecessary Doctrine of Necessaries," Note, *Michigan Law Review* 82 [June 1984]: 1770–1774).

10. Richard A. Chused, "Late Nineteenth Century Married Women's Property Law: Reception of the Early Married Women's Property Acts by Courts and Legislatures," *American Journal of Legal History* 29, no. 1 (1985): 1409–1410.

11. Evan Roberts, "Women's Rights and Women's Labor: Married Women's Property Laws and Labor Force Participation, 1860–1900," paper presented at the Economic History Association Annual Meeting, Pittsburgh, PA, September 14–16, 2006, 16, table 1, available at http://users.pop.umn .edu/~eroberts/eha2006.pdf (accessed July 1, 2008); Joan Hoff, *Law, Gender, and Injustice: A Legal History of U.S. Women* (New York: New York University Press, 1991), 127–135 and appendix I.

12. For example, Norma Basch, *In the Eyes of the Law: Women, Marriage, and Property in Nineteenth-Century New York* (Ithaca, NY: Cornell University Press, 1982); Carol Shammas, "Re-Assessing the Married Women's Property Acts," *Journal of Women's History* 6, no. 1 (Spring 1994): 9–30; Sara L.

Zeigler, "Uniformity and Conformity: Regionalism and Adjudication of the Married Women's Property Acts," *Polity* 28, no. 4 (Summer 1996): 467–495.

13. Reva B. Siegel, "The Modernization of Marital Status Law: Adjudicating Wives' Right to Earnings, 1860–1930," *The Georgetown Law Journal* 82 (1994): 2206–2207.

14. Katherine Silbaugh, "Turning Labor into Love: Housework and the Law," *Northwestern University Law Review* 91 (1996): 26. Another way to frame the difference, as Paulette Kidder does, is to characterize the exchanges of goods and services in public and private spheres as dominated by different logics, that of a market economy versus that of a gift economy, respectively (Paulette Kidder, "Gift Exchange and Justice in Families," *Journal of Social Philosophy* 32, no. 2 [Summer 2001]: 161–170). Kidder's analysis draws on Lewis Hyde's distinction between gift and market exchange. Interestingly, Hyde says that in a gift economy, the giver is obligated to give and the intended receiver is obligated to accept the gift and to reciprocate, which parallels the obligatory nature of status duties (Lewis Hyde, *The Gift: The Erotic Life of Property* [New York: Vintage Books, 1983], 8).

15. Grant v. Green, 41 Iowa 88 (Supreme Court of Iowa, 1875), 88.

16. Ibid., 91, 92.

17. Frame v. Frame, 36 S.W.2d 152 (Supreme Court of Texas, 1931), 154.

18. Bohanan v. Maxwell, 181 N.W. 683 (Supreme Court of Iowa, 1921); In re: Estate of Sonnicksen, 73 P.2d 643 (Court of Appeals of California, 1937), 479. See also Brooks v. Brooks, 119 P.2d 970 (Court of Appeals of California, 1941); and Luther v. National Bank of Commerce, 2 Wash.2d 470 (Supreme Court of Washington, 1940) for similar rulings.

19. Foxworthy v. Addams, 124 S.W. 381 (Court of Appeals of Kentucky, 1910), 383.

20. Coleman v. Burr, 45 Am. Rep. 160 (Court of Appeals of New York, 1883), 26.

21. Brooks v. Brooks, 350.

22. Miller v. Miller, 35 N.W. 464 (Supreme Court of Iowa, 1889), 183.

23. Coleman v. Burr, 22.

24. Ibid. 29.

25. Bohanan v. Maxwell, 687.

26. Relevant cases include Mason v. Dunbar, 5 N.W. 432 (Supreme Court of Michigan, 1880); Carver v. Wagner, 64 N.Y.S. 747 (Supreme Court of New York, 1900); Johnson v. Tait, 160 N.Y.S. 1000 (Supreme Court of New York, 1916); Bishop v. Haydon, 130 Iowa 250 (Supreme Court of Iowa, 1906); In re Estate of Kleinhesselink, 230 Iowa 1090 (Supreme Court of Iowa, 1941); In re: Talty, 5 N.W.2d 584 (Supreme Court of Iowa, 1942).

27. Borelli v. Brusseau, 12 Cal. App. 4th 647 (Court of Appeals of California, 1993), 649, 654.

28. Ryan v. Dockery, 134 Wis. 431 (Supreme Court of Wisconsin, 1908), 433.

29. In Re: Lord, 602 P.2d 1030 (Supreme Court of New Mexico, 1979), 1031, 1032.

30. Ryan v. Dockery, 432.

31. This principle was enunciated in Filer v. New York Central Railroad, 49 N.Y.47 (Court of Appeals of New York, 1872), 49; Blaechinska v. Howard Mission and Home for Little Wanderers, 29 N.E. 755 (Court of Appeals of New York, 1892), 757; Worley v. Gaston et al., 80 S.E.2d 304 (Supreme Court of Georgia, 1954), 306–307.

32. James M. Porter, "Husband and Wife: Right of Wife to Sue for Loss of Consortium Due to Negligent Injury to Husband," *Michigan Law Review* 55, no. 5 (March 1957): 721–724, esp. 721–722.

33. Mewhirter v. Hatten, 42 Iowa 288 (Supreme Court of Iowa, 1875), 291.

34. Mewhirter v. Hatten, 291, 292–293.

35. Metropolitan St. R.R. v. Johnson, 91 Ga. 466 (Supreme Court of Georgia, 1893), 471–472.

36. Denver Consolidated Tramway v. Riley, 14 Colo. App. 132 (Court of Appeals of Colorado, 1899), 140.

37. Meek v. Pacific Electric Railway Company, 175 Cal. 53 (Supreme Court of California, 1917), 56.

38. Gist v. French, 136 Cal. App. 2d 247 (Court of Appeals of California, 1955), 255–256.

39. Hitaffer v. Argonne, 183 F.2d. 811 (U.S. Court of Appeal, District of Columbia Circuit, 1950), 819.

40. "The Law in North American Legal Systems, (a) The United States. Action for Loss of Consortium," in *The Law Relating to Loss of Consortium and Loss of Services of a Child*, chapter 4 (Legal Reform Commission of Ireland, March, 2002), 29, available at http://www.lawreform.ie/publications/data/volume1/lrc_9.html-05 Mar 2002 (accessed February 7, 2007).

41. Price V. Fishback and Shawn Everett Kantor, "The Adoption of Workers' Compensation in the United States, 1900–1930," *Journal of Law and Economics* 41, no. 2 (October 1998): 320, table 2.

42. Christopher Howard, "Workers' Compensation, Federalism, and the Heavy Hand of History," *Studies in American Political Development* 16 (Spring 2002): 31.

43. Ibid., 32.

44. Fishback and Kanter, "The Adoption of Workers' Compensation," 316–317.

45. Ibid., 308–311.

46. Howard, "Workers' Compensation," 32–33.

47. "Workmen's Compensation Acts—Recovery by Wife for Nursing Services," *Harvard Law Review* 39, no. 8 (June 1926), 1105.

48. Galway v. Doody Steel Erecting Company, 103 Conn. 431 (Court of Error, First Judicial District, Connecticut, 1925), 435–436.

49. Claus v. Devere, 120 Neb. 812 (Supreme Court of Nebraska, 1931), 818. See also Bituminous Casualty Corp. v. Wilbanks, 23 S.E.2d 519 (Court of Appeals of Georgia, 1942); Meister v. E.W. Edwards, 37 N.Y.S.2d 56 (Supreme Court of New York, 1942); Coates v. Warren Hotel, 11 A.2d 436 (New Jersey Department of Labor, Workmen's Compensation Bureau, 1940).

50. Graf v. Montgomery Ward, 49 N.W.2d 797 (Supreme Court of Minnesota, 1951), 495.

51. Examples include two Missouri cases, Daugherty v. City of Monett, 192 S.W.2d (Court of Appeals of Missouri, 1946) and Collins v. Reed Harlin Grocery, 230 S.W.2d 880 (Springfield Court of Appeals, 1950), and a California case, California Casualty Indemnity Exchange v. Industrial Accident Commission, 190 P.2d 990 (Court of Appeals of California, 1948).

52. California Casualty Indemnity Exchange v. Industrial Accident Commission, 420.

53. Klaplac's Case, 242 N.E.2d (Supreme Judicial Court of Massachusetts, 1968), 47, footnote 2.

54. Warren Trucking Company v. Chandler, 277 S.E. 488 (Supreme Court of Virginia, 1981), 1116; see also Ross v. Northern States Power, 442 N.W.2d 296 (Supreme Court of Minnesota, 1989); St. Clair v. County of Grant, 797 P.2d 993 (Court of Appeals of New Mexico, 1990).

55. Kraemer v. Downey, 852 P.2d 1286 (Court of Appeals of Colorado, 1992), 1289. Other cases in which courts credited "on call" hours include Standard Blasting v. Hayman, 476 S.2d 1385 (Florida Appeals Court, 1985); Brown v. Eller, 314 N.W.2d 685 (Appeals Court of Michigan, 1981); Texas Employers Insurance v. Choate, 664 S.W.2d (Court of Appeals of Texas, 1982); Close v. Superior Excavating, Opinion no. 94–95WC (State of Vermont Department of Labor and Industries, 1995).

56. Jerome v. Farmers Produce Exchange, 797 S.W.2d 565 (Court of Appeals of Missouri, 1990), 568, 570.

57. Teague v. C. J. Chemical, 935 S.W.2d 605 (Court of Appeals of Arkansas, 1996); Standard Blasting & Coating v. Hayman, 476 So.2d 1385 (Court of Appeals of Florida, 1985); St. Clair v. County of Grant, 797 P.2d 993 (Court of Appeals of New Mexico, 1990); Transport Insurance Co. v. Polk, 400 S.W.2d 881 (Supreme Court of Texas, 1966); Close v. Superior Excavating, Opinion no. 94–95WC.

58. The 2008 Florida Statutes, Title XXI Labor, Chapter 440, Workers' Compensation, Section 440.13, (b), 1, 2 and 3, available at http://www.flsenate

.gov/Statutes/index.cfm?App_mode=Display_Statute&Search_String=& URL=Ch0440/SEC13.HTM&Title=-%3E2008-%3ECh0440-%3ESection %2013#0440.13 (accessed July 23, 2008). It appears that paragraphs 1 and 3 establish contradictory standards for caregivers who remain employed, at either minimum wage or at the community rate for such services, viz.:

1. If the family member is not employed or if the family member is employed and is providing attendant care services during hours that he or she is not engaged in employment, the per-hour value equals the federal minimum hourly wage.
2. If the family member is employed and elects to leave that employment to provide attendant or custodial care, the per-hour value of that care equals the per-hour value of the family member's former employment, not to exceed the per-hour value of such care available in the community at large. A family member or a combination of family members providing nonprofessional attendant care under this paragraph may not be compensated for more than a total of 12 hours per day.
3. If the family member remains employed while providing attendant or custodial care, the per-hour value of that care equals the per-hour value of the family member's employment, not to exceed the per-hour value of such care available in the community at large.

59. Supervising or giving cues to a person so he or she can perform tasks him- or herself has also been allowable since 1999; see Allen J. LeBlanc, Christine Tonner, and Charlene Harrington, "State Medicaid Programs Offering Personal Care Services," *Health Care Financing Review* 22, no. 4 (Summer 2001): 155.
60. "States' Requirements for Medicaid-Funded Personal Care Attendants," Office of the Inspector General, Department of Health and Human Services, October 2006, available at oig.hhs.gov/oei/reports/oei-07-05-00250. pdf (accessed June 20, 2008).
61. Department of Human Resources v. Williams, 202 S.E.2d 504 (Court of Appeals of Georgia, 1993).
62. Vincent v. State of California, 22 Cal. App. 3d 566 (Court of Appeals of California, 1971).
63. In 1981 federal legislation established a second program that offers some support for personal care services, the Home and Community Based Service Waivers, which gives states the option of providing home- and community-based services as an alternative to institutionalization. This program sets limits on how many individuals can receive services under the waiver, and it is difficult to assess the extent to which the program

offers personal care; see Le Blanc, Tonner, and Harrington, "State Medicaid Programs Offering Personal Care Services," 157.

64. "Benefits by Service: Personal Care Services (October 2004)," The Kaiser Commission on Medicaid and the Uninsured, available at http://www.kff.org/medicaid/benefits/service.jsp?gr=off&nt=on&so=0&tg=0&yr=2&cat=1&sv=28 (accessed January 21, 2007).

65. 42 C.F.R. § 440. 167, available at http://www.access.gpo.gov/nara/cfr/waisidx_02/42cfr440_02.html (accessed July 23, 2008).

66. Debi Waterstone, Taewoon Kang, Cristina Flores, Candace Howes, Charlene Harrington, and Robert Newcomer, *California's In-Home Supportive Services Program: Who Is Served?* (San Francisco: Center for Personal Assistance Services, University of California, San Francisco, 2004), available at http://www.pascenter.org/publications/publication_home.php?id=73PAS (accessed July 23, 2009), 4, 8.

67. Ibid. A chart comparing provisions of the three programs (Medical, Independence-Plus Waiver, and Residual) is available at www.disabilityrightsca.org/pubs/547001-App-J.pdf (accessed July 23, 2009). Robert Newcomer and Taewoon Kang, *Analysis of the California In-Home Supportive Services (IHSS) Plus Waiver Demonstration Program,* Report for the U.S. Department of Health and Human Services (July 2008), xvi, available at http://aspe.hhs.gov/daltcp/reports/2008/IHSSPlus.pdf (accessed July 24, 2009).

68. Pamela Doty, A. E. Benjamin, Ruth E. Matthias, and Todd M. Frank, *In-Home Support Services for the Elderly and Disabled: A Comparison of Client-Directed and Professional Management Models of Service Delivery,* Non Technical Summary Report, U.S. Department of Health and Human Services, April 1999, available at http://www.aspe.hhs.gov/taltcp/reports/ihss.htm (accessed January 25, 2007).

69. Ibid.

70. Martin Kitchener, Micky Willmott, Alice Wong, and Charlene Harrington, *Home and Community-Based Services: Medical Research and Demonstration Waivers* (San Francisco: Center for Personal Assistance Services, University of California, San Francisco, November, 2006), available at http://www.pascenter.org/demo_waivers/index.php (accessed January 25, 2007).

71. Laura L. Summer and Emily S. Ihara, *The Medicaid Personal Care Services Benefit: Practices in States That Offer the Optional State Plan Benefit* (Washington, DC: AARP Policy Institute, August 2005), 15, available at http://www.aarp.org/research/assistance/medicaid/2005_11_medicaid.html (accessed February 28, 2007).

72. Jae Kennedy and Simi Litvak, *Case Studies of Six State Personal Assistance Programs* (World Institute on Disability Research and Training Center on

Public Policy in Independent Living, December 1991), 19, available at http://
aspe.hhs.gov/daltcp/Reports/casestud.htm (accessed July 3, 2008). The authors note, "The exclusion of all family providers apparently caused particular problems for Native American consumers, who have a strong tradition of family support. Many of these consumers simply dropped off the
rolls" (19).

73. "Medicaid Personal Care Program," available at http://dhmh.state.md.us/
mma/longtermcare/html/Medicaid%20Personal%20Care.htm (accessed
January 21, 2007).

74. Kennedy and Litvak, *Case Studies of Six States*, 77.

75. Dade v. Anderson, 439 S.E.2d 353 (Supreme Court of Virginia, 1994), 6;
Paraprofessional Healthcare Institute, *State Chartbook for Personal and
Home Care Aides, 1999–2006,* prepared for Personal Assistance Services of
California, San Francisco (July 2008), available at http://www.pascenter.
org/publications/publication_home.php?id=857&focus=PAS%20Center
%20Publications (accessed August 20, 2008).

76. Janice M. Keefe and Pamela J. Fancey, *Financial Compensation versus Community Supports: An Analysis of the Effects on Caregivers and Care Receivers,*
Final Report (Health Canada, 1998), 28, available at http://www.members
.shaw.ca/bsalisbury/Financial%20Compensation%20versus%20Commu-
nity%20Supports.rtf (accessed January 23, 2008).

5. Paid Caring in the Home

1. Steven Greenhouse, "Day in Court for Queens Home-Care Aide," *New York
Times,* April 17, 2007.

2. Ibid.

3. Evelyn Nakano Glenn, *Unequal Freedom: How Race and Gender Shaped
American Citizenship and Labor* (Cambridge, MA: Harvard University Press,
2002), 240–242.

4. Sir William Blackstone, *Commentaries on the Laws of England* (London,
1765), Book 1, The Rights of Persons, Chapter the Fourteenth: Of Master
and Servant; Chapter the Fifteenth: Of Husband and Wife; Chapter the
Sixteenth, Of Parent and Child; Chapter the Seventeenth, Of Guardian
and Ward; The Avalon Project, Yale Law School, available at http://avalon
.law.yale.edu/subject_menus/blackstone.asp (accessed March 12, 2009).
Blackstone was cited frequently by American newspapers in the 1790s, a
critical period for the creation of state constitutions and the establishment
of legal norms. His conception of four hierarchies in household relations
was further codified by the first American professor of law, Tapping Reeve,
in his 1816 volume *The Law of Baron and Femme; of Parent and Child; of*

Guardian and Ward; of Master and Servant; and of the Powers of Courts of Chancer. Reeve's book was reissued in revised editions throughout the nineteenth century. See Holly Brewer, "The Transformation of Domestic Law," in Michael Grossberg and Christopher L. Tomlins, eds., *The Cambridge History of American Law,* vol. 1 (Cambridge: Cambridge University Press, 2008), 288–289.

5. Many social historians have posited a connection between social and economic change and the elaboration of the ideology of separate spheres in the nineteenth century, including Nancy Cott, *Bonds of Womanhood: "Woman's Sphere" in New England, 1780–1835* (New Haven, CT: Yale University Press, 1977), 64–70; Carl N. Degler, *At Odds: Women and the Family in America from the Revolution to the Present* (New York: Oxford University Press, 1980), 8–9, 26–29; Christopher Lasch, *Haven in a Heartless World: The Family Besieged* (New York: Basic Books, 1977, esp. 6–8 on the development of the contrasting visions of home and market). For a review of the historiography on separate spheres, see Linda K. Kerber, "Separate Spheres, Female Worlds, Women's Place: The Rhetoric of Women's History," in Cathy N. Davidson and Jessamyn Hatcher, eds., *No More Separate Spheres! A Next Wave American Studies Reader* (Durham, NC: Duke University Press, 2002), 29–65.

6. David Roediger, *The Wages of Whiteness: Race and the Making of the American Working Class* (London: Verso, 1991), 54.

7. Robert J. Steinfeld, *The Invention of Free Labor: The Employment Relation in English and American Law and Culture, 1350–1870* (Chapel Hill: University of North Carolina Press, 1991), 143–146.

8. Evelyn Nakano Glenn, "Racial Ethnic Women's Labor: The Intersection of Race, Gender, and Class Oppression," *Review of Radical Political Economy* 17, no. 3 (Fall 1985): 89–90, 95–96.

9. Amy Dru Stanley, *From Bondage to Contract: Wage Labor, Marriage, and the Market in the Age of Slave Emancipation* (New York: Cambridge University Press, 1998); Brewer, "The Transformation of Domestic Law," 291; Christopher Tomlins, "Subordination, Authority, Law: Subjects in Labor History," *International Labor and Working-Class History* 47 (March 1995): 78–80.

10. Karen Orren, *Belated Feudalism: Labor, the Law, and Liberal Development in the United States* (New York: Cambridge University Press, 1991), 15–19, 211–215; Robert J. Steinfeld, *Coercion, Contract, and Free Labor* (Cambridge: Cambridge University Press, 2001), 253–289.

11. Lochner v. New York, 198 U.S. 45 (1905); Coppage v. Kansas, 236 U.S. 1 (Supreme Court of the United States, 1915). Another oft-cited precedent at the state level was an earlier case, Godcharles v. Wigeman, 113 Pa. 431

(1886), in which a Pennsylvania Court overturned a state law prohibiting payment of wages in kind instead of cash. See also Arthur F. McAvoy, "Freedom of Contract, Labor, and the Administrative State," in Harry N. Scheiber, ed., *The State and Freedom of Contract* (Stanford, CA: Stanford University Press, 1998), 210–214.

12. Muller v. Oregon, 208 U.S. 412 (1908); for a history of protective labor legislation for women, see Alice Kessler-Harris, *In Pursuit of Equity: Women, Men and the Quest for Economic Citizenship* (New York: Oxford University Press, 2002), 30–33.

13. George O. Butler, "The Black Worker in Industry, Agriculture, Domestic and Personal Service," *Journal of Negro Education* 8, no. 3 (July 1939): 426; Jean Collier Brown, *The Negro Woman Worker,* Women's Bureau Bulletin no. 165 (Washington, DC: Government Printing Office, 1938), 3.

14. Adkins v. Children's Hospital, 261 U.S. 525 (Supreme Court of the United States, 1923).

15. Text and audio of Roosevelt's First Inaugural Address, available at http://historymatters.gmu.edu/d/5057/ (accessed March 18, 2008).

16. National Industrial Recovery Act, transcript available at http://www.ourdocuments.gov/doc.php?doc=66&page=transcript (accessed March 19, 2008); Leverett Lyon, *The National Recovery Administration: An Analysis and Appraisal* (Washington, DC: Brookings Institution, 1935). For a quick overview, see Barbara Alexander, "National Recovery Administration," EH.Net Encyclopedia, edited by Robert Whaples, August 14, 2001, available at http://eh.net/encyclopedia/article/alexander.nra (accessed March 19, 2008).

17. Schecter Poultry Corp. v. United States, 295 U.S. 495 (Supreme Court of the United States, 1935).

18. Section 7a reads, "Every code of fair competition, agreement, and license approved, prescribed, or issued under this title shall contain the following conditions: (1) That employees shall have the right to organize and bargain collectively through representatives of their own choosing, and shall be free from the interference, restraint, or coercion of employers of labor, or their agents, in the designation of such representatives or in self-organization or in other concerted activities for the purpose of collective bargaining or other mutual aid or protection; (2) that no employee and no one seeking employment shall be required as a condition of employment to join any company union or to refrain from joining, organizing, or assisting a labor organization of his own choosing; and (3) that employers shall comply with the maximum hours of labor, minimum rates of pay, and other conditions of employment, approved or prescribed by the President."

19. National Labor Relations Act, 29 U.S.C. §§ 151–169; Abner J. Mivka, "The Changing Role of the Wagner Act in the American Labor Movement," *Stanford Law Review* 38, no. 4 (April 1986): 1124–1127.

20. Suzanne Mettler, *Dividing Citizens: Gender and Federalism in New Deal Public Policy* (Ithaca, NY: Cornell University Press, 1998), 179, 182; Kessler-Harris, *In Pursuit of Equity*, 101–105; 29 C.F.R. § 531.27.

21. Suzanne B. Mettler, "Federalism, Gender, and the Fair Labor Standards Act of 1938," *Polity* 26, no. 4 (Summer 1994): 642–643.

22. National Labor Relations Board v. Jones & Laughlin Steel Corporation, 301 U.S. 1 (Supreme Court of the United States, 1937); United States v. Darby Lumber Co. 312 U.S. 100 (Supreme Court of the United States, 1941).

23. Orren, *Belated Feudalism*, 15–19; Richard A. Brisbin Jr., *A Strike Like No Other Strike: Law and Resistance during the Pittston Coal Strike of 1989–1990* (Baltimore, MD: Johns Hopkins University Press, 2002), 28–32.

24. Katherine Silbaugh, "Turning Labor into Love: Housework and the Law," *Northwestern University Law Review* 91, no. 1 (Fall 1996): 74.

25. Eileen Boris and Premilla Nadasen, "Domestic Workers Organize!" *WorkingUSA* 11, no. 4 (December 2008): 413–437; Tera W. Hunter, *To 'Joy My Freedom: Southern Black Women's Lives and Labors after the Civil War* (Cambridge, MA: Harvard University Press, 1998), 74–97; Elizabeth L. O'Leary, *From Morning to Night: Domestic Service in Maymont House and the Gilded Age South* (Charlottesville: University of Virginia Press, 2003), 107–108; Teresa L. Amott and Julie A. Matthaei, *Race, Gender and Work: A Multi-Cultural Economic History of Women in the United States,* rev. ed. (Boston: South End Press, 1999), 171.

26. Silbaugh, "Turning Labor into Love," 74.

27. State v. Cooper, 285 N.W. 903 (Minnesota 1939), 905.

28. Ankh Services, Inc., 243 N.L.R.B. 478 (1979), 480.

29. Phyllis Palmer, "Outside the Law: Agricultural and Domestic Workers under the Fair Labor Standards Act 1938–1974," *Journal of Policy History* 7, no. 4 (1995): 416–440; Vivien Hart, "Minimum Wage Policy and Constitutional Inequality: The Paradox of the Fair Labor Standards Act of 1938," *Journal of Policy History* 1 (1989): 319–343.

30. Mettler, *Dividing Citizens,* 186–187, 194–195.

31. Civil Rights Act of 1964—CRA—Title VII—Equal Employment Opportunities, 42 U.S. Code chapter 21; Kessler-Harris, *In Pursuit of Equity,* 234; Dorothy Sue Cobble, *The Other Women's Movement: Workplace Justice and Social Justice in Modern America* (Princeton, NJ: Princeton University Press, 2006), 166–167, 220.

32. *Congressional Record—House,* June 6, 1973, FLSA Amendments of 1973 (Washington, DC: U.S. Government Printing Office, 1973), 296.

33. *Congressional Record—House,* June 5, 1973, FLSA Amendments of 1973 (Washington, DC: U.S. Government Printing Office, 1973), 264, 279.

34. Ibid., 258–259.

35. Ibid., 249–250.

36. Palmer, "Outside the Law," 417–418.

37. *Congressional Record—House,* June 5, 1973, FLSA Amendments of 1973, 266.

38. *Congressional Record—House,* June 6, 1973, FLSA Amendments of 1973, 282.

39. Ibid., 279.

40. *Congressional Record—Senate,* July 19, 1973, FLSA Amendments of 1973 (Washington, DC: U.S. Government Printing Office, 1973), 958.

41. Ibid., 951.

42. Ibid.

43. "Minority Views of Messrs. Dominick, Taft, and Beall," FLSA 1974, 1, 599.

44. Subcommittee on Labor of the Committee on Labor and Public Welfare, United States Senate, *Legislative History of the Fair Labor Standards Amendments of 1974* (Washington, DC: Government Printing Office, 1976), II, 1823.

45. 29 C.F.R. 552.2 (Code of Federal Regulations Pertaining to ESA, U.S. Department of Labor, last revised 9/8/95).

46. Mr. Williams Report from Committee on Labor and Public Welfare, U.S. Senate, July 6, 1973 in re: FLSA Amendments of 1973.

47. *Congressional Record—Senate,* July 19, 1973, FLSA of 1973, 963.

48. Ibid., 973.

49. Statement on Signing the Fair Labor Standards Amendments of 1974, April 8, 1974, available at http://www.presidency.ucsb.edu/ws/index.php?pid=4169 (accessed July 13, 2008).

50. 29 CFR 552.109.

51. 29 CFR 552.6.

52. Wage and Hour Division, Employment Standards Administration, Labor, "Application of the Fair Labor Standards Act to Domestic Service: Notice of Proposed Rulemaking and Request for Comments," *Federal Register* 66, no. 13 (January 19, 2001): 5481–5489, available at http://www.sba.gov/advo/laws/comments/ddol01_0322.html (accessed August 16, 2008).

53. Transcript, Long Island Care at Home v. Coke, No. 06-593, in the Supreme Court of the United States, Oral Argument, April 16, 2007, The Oyez Project, available at http://www.oyez.org/cases/2000-2009/2006/2006_06_593 (accessed August 16, 2007); Long Island Care at Home v. Coke, Brief for Respondent; Long Island Care at Home v. Coke, Brief for Plaintiff, available at same site (accessed August 16, 2007).

54. Long Island Care at Home v. Coke, 462 F.3d 48 (2004); 126 S. Ct. 1189 (2006); 127 S. Ct. 853 (2007); list of amicus curiae briefs in Long Island Care at Home, Ltd. v. Coke, available at http://www.supremecourtus.gov/docket/06-593.htm (accessed August 16, 2008).

55. Transcript, Long Island Care at Home, Ltd. v. Coke, Oral Argument, available at http://www.oyez.org/cases/2000-2009/2006/2006_06_593/argument/; Coke v. Long Island Care at Home, 376 F.3d 118 (2004); Long Island Care at Home v. Coke, 376 F.3d 118 (2d Cir. 2004); Long Island Care at Home v. Coke, 126 S. Ct. 1189 (January 23, 2006); Long Island Care v. Coke, 127 S. Ct 853 (January 5, 2007); Greenhouse, "Day in Court for Queens Home-Care Aide," 1.

56. Long Island Care at Home v. Coke, 551 U.S. — (2007); Long Island Care at Home v. Coke, 462 F.3d 48 (2004).

57. Peggie R. Smith, "Regulating Paid Household Work: Class, Gender, Race, and Agendas of Reform," *American University Law Review* 48 (1999): 914.

58. B-1 visas described on U.S. Citizenship and Immigration Services' Web site, http://www.uscis.gov/propub/ProPubVAP.jsp?dockey=80abe45edac45083eb0d44706417c757 (accessed January 16, 2008).

59. From the Web site of the visa assistance firm Visapro, available at http://faq.visapro.com/G5-Visa-FAQ4.asp (accessed January 16, 2008).

60. Joy M. Zarembka, "Maid to Order," in Barbara Ehrenreich and Arlie Russell Hochschild, *Global Woman: Nannies, Maids, and Sex Workers in the New Economy* (New York: Henry Holt, 2004), 145.

61. U.S. Department of State Foreign Affairs Manual Volume 9—Visas, 9 Fam 41.21 N6.1–6.6, 4–9, available at www.state.gov/documents/organization/87174.pdf (accessed July 20, 2009); "Hidden in the Home: Abuse of Domestic Workers with Special Visas in the United States," *Human Rights Watch* 13, no. 1 (June 1, 2001): 22, available at http://www.hrw.org/legacy/reports/2001/usadom/ (accessed August 1, 2009).

62. "Nanny Protection Bill Becomes Law," available at http://www.casademaryland.org/index.php?option=com_content&view=article&id=388:07232008&catid=42:news&Itemid=127 (accessed September 21, 2009).

63. "NY Domestic Workers Bill of Rights," available at http://www.domesticworkersunited.org/campaigns.php (accessed September 21, 2009). The New York State Assembly passed a watered-down version on June 22, 2009, report available at http://assembly.state.ny.us/leg/?bn=A01470 (accessed September 21, 2009). The State Senate had not yet voted on the proposed bill as of mid-December 2009.

64. Campaign announced at http://www.afscmeinfocenter.org/2009/03/rights-begin-at-home-defending-domestic-workers-rights-in-california.htm (accessed September 21, 2009).

65. Douglas Martin, "Evelyn Coke, Home Care Aide Who Fought Pay Rule, Is Dead at 74," *New York Times,* August 10, 2009, available at http://www .nytimes.com/2009/08/10/nyregion/10coke.html?_r=2&hpw (accessed August 16, 2009).

6. Neoliberalism and Globalization

1. U.S. Department of Health and Human Services, *The Future Supply of Long Term Care Workers in Relation to the Aging Baby Boom Generation: Report to Congress* (Washington, DC: Government Printing Office, 2003), 4.

2. William J. Scanlon, Testimony of Director, Health Care Issues, U.S. General Accounting Office, in *Nursing Workforce: Recruitment and Retention of Nurses and Nurse Aides Is a Growing Concern* (Washington, DC: General Accounting Office, 2001), 10.

3. Institute for Health and Aging, *Chronic Care in America* (San Francisco, CA: University of California, San Francisco, 1996), 193; Nora Super, *Who Will Be There to Care? The Growing Gap between Caregiver Supply and Demand,* National Health Policy Forum Background Paper (Washington, DC: The George Washington University, January 23, 2002), 3, citing National Family Caregivers Association, "Family Caregiving Statistics" (Kensington, MD, 2000).

4. *Grandparents Living with Grandchildren: 2000,* Census 2000 Brief (Washington, DC: Government Printing Office, October 2003), 3–4, 8–9; Esme Fuller-Thomson and Meredith Minkler, "American Grandparents Providing Extensive Child Care to Their Grandchildren: Prevalence and Profile," *The Gerontologist* 41, no. 2 (April 2001): 201–209; Meredith Minkler and Esme Fuller-Thomson, "The Health of Grandparents Raising Grandchildren: Results of a National Study," *American Journal of Public Health* 89, no. 9 (September 1999): 1384–1389; Linda M. Burton, "Black Grandparents Rearing Children of Drug-Addicted Parents: Stressors, Outcomes, and Social Service Needs," *The Gerontologist* 32, no. 6 (1992): 744–751.

5. Nona Glazer, *Women's Paid and Unpaid Labor: The Work Transfer in Health Care and Retailing* (Philadelphia: Temple University Press, 1993).

6. William Ruddick, "Transforming Homes and Hospitals," in John D. Arras, ed., *Bringing the Hospital Home: Ethical and Social Implications of High-Tech Home Care* (Baltimore, MD: Johns Hopkins University Press, 1995), 186.

7. Abigail Zuger, "Arming Unsung Heroes of Health Care," *New York Times,* October 26, 1999, available at http://www.nytimes.com/1999/10/26/health/ essay-arming-unsung-heroes-of-health-care.html?scp=14&sq= Abigail+Zuger+Essay&st=nyt (accessed January 18, 2008); National Alliance for Caregiving and AARP, *Caregiving in the U.S.: Findings from the*

National Caregiver Survey (2004), 8–9, available at http://www.caregiving
.org/pubs/data.htm.

8. Rosalie Kane, "High Tech Home Care in Context: Organization, Quality, and Ethical Ramifications," in John D. Arras, ed., *Bringing the Hospital Home: Ethical and Social Implications of High-Tech Home Care* (Baltimore, MD: Johns Hopkins University Press, 1995), 197.

9. Nancy Guberman, Eric Gagnon, Denyse Cote, Claude Gilbert, Nichole Thivierge, and Marielle Tremblay, "How the Trivialization of the Demands of High Tech Care in the Home Is Turning Family Members into Para-Medical Personnel," *Journal of Family Issues* 26, no. 2 (March 2005): 249.

10. Pascale Lehoux, J. Saint-Arnaud, and L. Richard, "The Use of Technology in the Home: What Manuals Say and Sell vs. What Patients Face and Fear," *Sociology of Health & Illness* 26, no. 5 (2004): 630–631.

11. Cameron Macdonald, "The Home as Hospital: A Pilot Study Investigating the Consequences of High-Tech Home Care for Patients and Their Families," paper presented at the Intimate Labors Conference, University of California, Santa Barbara, October 4–6, 2007, 6.

12. Ibid., 4.

13. Emily Abel, *Hearts of Wisdom: American Women Caring for Kin, 1850–1940* (Cambridge, MA: Harvard University Press, 2000), 44–46.

14. Nel Noddings, "Moral Obligation or Moral Support for High-Tech Home Care?" in John D. Arras, ed., *Bringing the Hospital Home: Ethical and Social Implications of High-Tech Home Care* (Baltimore, MD: Johns Hopkins University Press, 1995), 155.

15. Macdonald, "The Home as Hospital," 3–4.

16. Ibid., 4.

17. John D. Arras and Nancy Neveloff Dubler, "Introduction: Ethical and Social Implications of High-Tech Home Care," in John D. Arras, ed., *Bringing the Hospital Home: Ethical and Social Implications of High-Tech Home Care* (Baltimore, MD: Johns Hopkins University Press, 1995), 6.

18. Pascale Lehoux, "Patients' Perspectives on High-Tech Home Care: A Qualitative Inquiry into the User-Friendliness of Four Technologies," *BMC Health Services Research* 4 (2004): 6 of 9, available at http://www.biomed central.com/content/pdf/1472-6963-4-28.pdf (accessed January 16, 2009).

19. Guberman et al., "The Trivialization of Demands of High-Tech Care," 268.

20. Arras and Dubler, "Introduction," 21.

21. Robert Frost, "The Death of the Hired Hand," in *North of Boston* (New York: Henry Holt, 1917), 20.

22. Carol Levine, "Home Sweet Hospital: The Nature and Limits of Private Responsibilities for Home Health Care," *Journal of Aging and Health* 11, no. 3 (August 1999): 351.

23. Martha F. Davis, *Brutal Need: Lawyers and the Welfare Rights Movement, 1960–1973* (New Haven, CT: Yale University Press, 1993), 56; Felicia Kornbluh, *The Battle for Welfare Rights: Politics and Poverty in Modern America* (Philadelphia: University of Pennsylvania Press, 2007), 69; Charles Murray, *Losing Ground: American Social Policy, 1950–1980* (New York: Basic Books, 1984); Lawrence Mead, *Beyond Entitlement: The Social Obligations of Citizenship* (New York: Basic Books, 1986).

24. Kornbluh, *Welfare Rights,* 89–91; Personal Responsibility and Work Opportunity Reconciliation Act of 1996, Public Law No. 104-193, 110 Stat. 2105 (1996) (codified as amended at 42 U.S.C. 601–617).

25. Joanne L. Goodwin, "'Employable Mothers' and 'Suitable Work': A Re-valuation of Welfare and Wage-Earning for Women in the Twentieth Century United States," *Journal of Social History* 29, no. 2 (Winter 1995): 255.

26. Joanne L. Goodwin, *Gender and the Politics of Welfare Reform: Mothers' Pensions in Chicago, 1911–1929* (Chicago: University of Chicago Press, 1997), 129; Linda Gordon, *Pitied but Not Entitled: Single Mothers and the History of Welfare, 1890–1935* (New York: The Free Press, 1994), 49–50.

27. Goodwin, *Gender and the Politics of Welfare Reform,* 161. For example, in 1919, only two states allowed pensions to unmarried mothers. See Carolyn M. Moehling, "Mother's Pensions and Female Headship," 6, draft paper available at http://www.econ.yale.edu/seminars/labor/lap02/Moehling-021004.pdf (accessed December 15, 2009).

28. Gwendolyn Mink, *The Wages of Motherhood: Inequality in the Welfare State, 1917–1942* (Ithaca, NY: Cornell University Press, 1995), 49–50.

29. Goodwin, "'Employable Mothers' and 'Suitable Work,'" 259; Social Security Act (Act of 1935, Title IV, Sec. 403).

30. Mink, *The Wages of Motherhood,* 131–132.

31. Grace Abbott, *From Relief to Social Security: The Development of the New Public Welfare Services and Their Administration* (Chicago: University of Chicago Press, 1941), 211.

32. Goodwin, "'Employable Mothers' and 'Suitable Work,'" 260.

33. Ibid., 261.

34. Lisa Levenstein, "From Innocent Children to Unwanted Migrants and Unwed Moms: Two Chapters in the Public Discourse on Welfare in the United States, 1960–1961," *Journal of Women's History* 11, no. 4 (2000): 13, 17.

35. Ibid., 25.

36. Ibid., 23.

37. Susan W. Blank and Barbara B. Blum, "A Brief History of Work Expectations for Welfare Mothers," *The Future of Children* 7, no. 1 (Spring 1997): 31.

38. Goodwin, "'Employable Mothers' and 'Suitable Work,'" 267–268.

39. Family Support Act of 1988, Public Law 100-485, 102 Stat. 2343 (October 13, 1988), codified in sections of 42 U.S.C.; Reagan signing statement, available at http://www.reagan.utexas.edu/archives/speeches/1988/101388a .htmJOBS program (accessed August 23, 2009).

40. LaDonna Pavetti, "The Challenge of Achieving High Work Participation Rates in Welfare Programs," Brookings Institution Policy Brief, Welfare Reform & Beyond, no. 31 (October 2004), 2, available at http://www.brookings .edu/es/wrb/publications/pb/pb31.pdf (accessed August 23, 2009).

41. Daniel T. Lichter and Rukamalie Jayakody, "Welfare Reform: How Do We Measure Success?" *Annual Review of Sociology* 28 (2002): 119; James P. Ziliak, David N. Figlio, Elizabeth E. Davis, and Laura S. Connolly, "Accounting for the Decline in AFDC Caseloads: Welfare Reform or Economic Growth?" *Journal of Human Resources* 35, no. 3 (2000): 570, 580, table 4.

42. Gregory Acs and Pamela Loprest, *Leaving Welfare: Employment and Well-Being of Families That Left Welfare in the Post-Entitlement Era* (Kalamazoo, MI: Upjohn Institute, 2004), 66, 67.

43. Nita Patel, "Work Force Development: Employment Retention and Advancement Under TANF," Technical Paper (Battle Creek, MI: W. K. Kellogg Foundation, n.d.), 1.

44. Sharon Parrott, "Welfare Recipients Who Find Jobs: What Do We Know about Their Employment and Earnings?" (Washington, DC: Center on Budget and Policy Priorities, 1998), 6, 10, 13, 19.

45. Pamela Loprest, "Families Who Left Welfare: Who Are They and How Are They Doing?" Discussion Paper (Washington, DC: Urban Institute, 1999), 11, available at http://www.urban.org/publications/310290.html (accessed August 16, 2008).

46. Parrott, "Welfare Recipients Who Find Jobs," 11.

47. Sharon Hayes, *Flat Broke with Children: Women in the Age of Welfare Reform* (Oxford: Oxford University Press, 2003), 25.

48. These studies are *Welfare Reform and Children Study,* which has carried out surveys and ethnographic studies in Boston, Chicago, and San Antonio (see project Web site at http://www.jhu.edu/~welfare); *Fragile Families and Child Well-Being Study* (Web site at http://www.nichd.nih.gov/ about/cpr/dbs/res_fragile.html); and *Project on Devolution and Urban Change* (Web site at http//www.mdrc.org/project_25_3.html) (all accessed December 15, 2009).

49. Women on welfare agree with the general public that welfare reform is good in that some people have taken advantage of entitlements to avoid responsibility. However, they also argue that many people need help and that they should get public assistance without being stigmatized.

50. P. Lindsay Chase-Lansdale, Robert A. Moffitt, Brenda J. Lohman, Andrew J. Cherlin, Rebekah Levine Coley, Laura D. Pittman, Jennifer Roff, and Elizabeth Votruba-Drzal, "Mothers' Transitions from Welfare to Work and the Well-Being of Preschoolers and Adolescents," *Science* 299 (March 7, 2003): 1551.

51. Laura Lein, Alan F. Benjamin, Monica McManus, and Kevin Roy, "Without a Net, Without a Job: What's a Mother to Do?" in Jane Henrici, ed., *Doing Without: Women and Work after Welfare Reform* (Tucson: University of Arizona Press, 2006), 24–25.

52. Ellen K. Scott, Andrew S. London, and Glenda Gross, "'I Try Not to Depend on Anyone but Me': Welfare-Reliant Women's Perspectives on Self-Sufficiency, Work, and Marriage," *Sociological Inquiry* 77, no. 4 (November 2007): 610–612.

53. Andrew S. London, Ellen K. Scott, Kathryn Edin, and Vicki Hunter, "Welfare Reform, Work-Family Tradeoffs, and Child Well-Being," *Family Relations* 53, no. 2 (2004): 154.

54. Lein et al., "Without a Net," 26.

55. Kevin M. Roy, Carolyn Y. Tubbs, and Linda M. Burton, "Don't Have No Time: Daily Rhythms and the Organization of Time for Low-Income Families," *Family Relations* 53, no. 2 (2004): 173.

56. London et al., "Welfare Reform," 154.

57. Chase-Lansdale et al., "Mothers' Transitions," 1550.

58. Carolyn Y. Tubbs, Kevin M. Roy, and Linda M. Burton, "Family Ties: Constructing Family Time in Low-Income Families," *Family Process* 44, no. 2 (2005): 84.

59. Roy et al., "Don't Have No Time," 174.

60. Tubbs, Roy, and Burton, "Family Ties," 86, 88.

61. Jodi Eileen Morris and Rebekah Levine Coley, "Maternal, Family, and Work Correlates of Role Strain in Low-Income Mothers," *Journal of Family Psychology* 188, no. 3 (2004): 424–432.

62. Laura Lein, "The Importance of Selection Factors: Evaluating the Impact of Employment on Family Well-Being in Families Transitioning from Welfare to Work," *Human Behavior in the Social Environment* 13, no. 1 (2006): 58.

63. Enid Kasser, *The Medicaid Personal Care Services Benefit: Practices in States That Offer the Optional State Plan Benefit* (Washington, DC: AARP, 2005), 9.

64. U.S. Department of Health and Human Services, Office of the Assistant Secretary for Planning and Evaluation, *Understanding Medicaid Home and Community Services: A Primer* (Washington, DC: Office of the Secretary, Department of Health and Human Services, October 2000), 13. The scope

of services under waivers can be quite extensive. According to this HHS report, "Services covered under waiver programs include case management, homemaker, home health aid, personal care, adult day health, habilitation, respite care, 'such other services requested by the state as the Secretary may approve,' and 'day treatment or other partial hospitalization services, psychosocial rehabilitation services, and clinic services (whether or not furnished in a facility) for individuals with chronic mental illness.'"

65. Wendy Fox-Grage, Barbara Coleman, and Marc Freiman, "Rebalancing: Ensuring Greater Access to Home and Community-Based Services," Fact Sheet (Washington, DC: AARP Public Policy Institute, 2006), 1, available at http://www.aarp.org/ppi (accessed June 7, 2008).

66. Bureau of Labor Statistics, *National Occupational Employment and Wage Estimates, May 2006* (Washington, DC: U.S. Department of Labor Bureau of Labor Statistics, May 2007), available at http://www.bls.gov/oes/current/oes_nat.htm#b00-0000 (accessed July 29, 2008).

67. Arlene Dohm and Lynn Shniper, "Occupational Employment Projections to 2016," *Monthly Labor Review* (Washington, DC: U.S. Department of Labor, November 2007), 94.

68. The Web site for Partners in Care features the following description of its services:

- Over 6,000 home health aides (HHAs), RNs and LPNs on staff
- All of our home health aides receive 30 hours of training over the state requirements
- We are a licensed and insured agency
- We have over 20 years of experience serving New Yorkers
- All of our home care aides must pass comprehensive drug tests, fingerprinting and criminal background checks
- We provide comprehensive in home services including companionship, private duty nursing, personal assistance, housekeeping, home health aides, PRI [Patient Review Instrument] assessments as well as geriatric care management
- We provide in home care, part time or full-time, live in care or congregate care at an assisted living facility or retirement community.

Indicating the transnational nature of the caring labor force in the United States, the six home health aides featured under "Our Outstanding Caregivers" are: Maria (a Russian immigrant), Rosa (originally from Puerto Rico), Veronica (African American), Hawanatu (from West Africa), Eleanor (Haitian), and Frankie (a male, from Puerto Rico). Descriptions are available at http://www.partnersincareny.org/a_index.html (accessed June 17, 2008).

69. See the Web site for Cooperative Home Care Associates at http://www
.chcany.org/; further description is listed on the National Clearinghouse
on the Direct Care Workforce Web site at http://www.directcareclearing
house.org/practices/r_pp_det.jsp?res_id=48910 (both accessed June 20,
2008).

70. Jane Gross, "New Options (and Risks) in Home Care for Elders," *New York
Times,* March 1, 2007. According to SeniorBridge's Web site: "All our Home
Health Aides and Companions are chosen based on the most rigorous and
selective process in the industry. The goal of our screening process is to
select only dedicated and outstanding people who hold caring as one of
their most important personal values. We recognize they are the foundation of the care we provide our clients. Our Home Health Aides all have
certificates in home health care. Their responsibilities are to assist the client with Activities of Daily Living and Instrumental Activities of Daily
Living, such as eating, bathing, dressing, providing medication reminders
and shopping for groceries. They make sure the client is comfortable and
without pain, enhancing their quality of life and comfort." SeniorBridge
Web site, http://www.seniorbridge.net/team-meet.shtml (accessed July 7,
2008). The HouseWorks Web site states that it is "A division of Solomont
Bailis Venture." Using the language of retail chains that call their sales
people "associates," HouseWorks says "All services are provided by experienced Home Care Associates who meet HouseWorks selective hiring standards. Associates providing personal care and skilled services are Certified Nursing Assistants or Certified Home Health Aides." It also notes that
it has established "preferred home care provider" status with several affluent senior residential communities, Beacon Hill Village in Boston, Cambridge Home in Cambridge, Massachusetts, and The Watergate Initiative
in Washington, D.C. The Web site of House Works is at http://www.house
-works.com/homeCare/index.htm (accessed July 7, 2008).

71. Information on Home Instead is found at its Web site, http://www.homein
stead.com/frandev/default.aspx (accessed July 8, 2008). On other pages of
its Web site, Home Instead claims: "Home Instead Senior Care franchise
owners have built successful and rewarding businesses by providing an
affordable solution for the elderly who prefer to remain at home for as long
as possible. Services (part-time, full-time and around-the-clock) are designed for seniors who need just a little help from a friend to live independently. Caregivers provide just that: a little help in the form of companionship, meal preparation, medication reminders, light housekeeping and
help with errands so that seniors from Toledo to Tokyo, Baltimore to Bris-
bane, Detroit to Dublin and Los Angeles to London can remain safely
and comfortably in their own homes." Another page designed to attract

franchisers states, "Home Instead Senior Care is one of the most affordable options in all of franchising. Total start-up costs range from $39,050–$52,050, including the initial franchise fee of $27,500 (US & Canada)." This URL is http://www.homeinstead.com/frandev/Lists/FAQLib/ShowFAQ.aspx (accessed July 8, 2008). Visiting Angel's Web site notes on its contact site: "Visiting Angels® / Senior Homecare By Angels® has established over 400 senior home care franchises in 47 states across the United States (and Canada). We advertise and market nationally for homecare client leads and distribute hundreds of home care client leads each week to our franchisees!" The contact page can be reached via Visiting Angel's franchise Web site at http://www.livingassistance.com/fran%20op.htm. Like many franchise operations, it maintains separate or interlinked Web sites for clients (http://www.visitingangels.com/default.asp) (both accessed July 8, 2008).

72. Gross, "New Options (and Risks) in Home Care for Elderly."
73. "Subcontracting," Home Health Care Reimbursement Work Group, 2009, available at http://www.health.state.ny.us/facilities/long_term_care/reimbursement/docs/2009-07-07_home_health_care_reimbursement_workgroup_meeting.pdf (accessed January 12, 2010); Gross, "New Options (and Risks in Home Care for Elderly)."
74. Ibid.
75. These observations stem from my own involvement in the gray market in searching for and finding home care for my mother.
76. "Julita" and all other names of workers are pseudonyms.
77. Rhonda J. V. Montgomery, Lyn Holley, Jerome Deichert, and Karl Kosloski, "A Profile of Home Care Workers from the 2000 Census: How It Changes What We Know," *Gerontologist* 45 (2005): 593–600. According to Montgomery et al., in 1999, 34 percent of home-care aides worked full-time year around.
78. William J. Scanlon, Testimony of Director, Health Care Issues, U.S. General Accounting Office, in *Nursing Workforce,* 21.
79. Montgomery et al., "A Profile of Home Care Workers from the 2000 Census," 596; Walter N. Leutz, "Immigration and the Elderly: Foreign-Born Workers in Long-Term Care," *Immigration Policy in Focus* 5, no. 12 (August 2007), 4. The category is made up of both Home Care Aides and Personal Care Aides and thus includes those who assist elderly or disabled individuals at home or in daytime non-residential facilities.
80. Annette Bernhardt, Siobhán McGrath, and James DeFilippis, *Unregulated Work in the Global City* (New York: Brennan Center for Justice, New York University School of Law, 2007), 36, available at http://nelp.3cdn.net/cc4d61e5942f9cfdc5_d6m6bgaq4.pdf (accessed August 20, 2008).
81. Ibid., 70.

82. Dawn Lyon, "The Organization of Care Work in Italy: Gender and Migrant Labor in the New Economy," *Indiana Journal of Global Legal Studies* 13, no. 1 (Winter 2006): 208.

83. Grace Chang, *Disposable Domestics: Immigrant Workers in the Global Economy* (Boston: South End Press, 2000), 123–124.

84. For in-depth studies of migration of women from the global south to fill the demand for caring labor in the global north, see Rhacel Salazar Parrenas, *Servants of Globalization: Women, Migration, and Domestic Work* (Palo Alto, CA: Stanford University Press, 2001); Pierrette Hondagneu-Sotelo, *Domestica: Immigrant Workers Cleaning and Caring in the Shadows of Affluence* (Berkeley: University of California Press, 2001); Pei-chia Lan, *Global Cinderellas: Migrant Domestics and Newly Rich Employers in Taiwan* (Durham, NC: Duke University Press, 2006); and Helma Lutz, ed., *Migration and Domestic Work: A European Perspective on a Global Theme* (Burlington, VT: Ashgate Publishing, 2008).

7. Creating a Caring Society

1. Joan Tronto, *Moral Boundaries: A Political Argument for an Ethic of Care* (New York: Routledge, 1993); Diemut Elisabet Bubeck, *Care, Gender, and Justice* (Oxford: Clarendon Press, 1995); Emily Abel and Margaret Nelson, eds., *Circles of Care* (Albany: State University of New York Press, 1990); Sara Ruddick, "Care as Labor and Relationship," in Joram G. Haber and Mark S. Halfon, eds., *Norms and Values: Essays on the Work of Virginia Held* (Lanham, MD: Rowman and Littlefield, 1998), 3–25.

2. Ruddick, "Care as Labor and Relationship," 11.

3. Ibid., 14; Tronto, *Moral Boundaries,* 135.

4. Barrie Thorne, "Pick-Up Time at Oakdale Elementary School: Work and Family from the Vantage Points of Children," in Rosanna Hertz and Nancy Marshall, eds., *Working Families: The Transformation of the American Home* (Berkeley: University of California Press, 2001), 354–376.

5. Barbara Hobson, "Solo Mothers, Social Policy Regimes, and the Logics of Gender," in Diane Sainsbury, ed., *Gendering Welfare States* (London: Sage Publications, 1994), 170–187; Francesca M. Cancian and Stacey J. Oliker, *Caring and Gender* (Thousand Oaks, CA: Pine Forge Press, 2000), 120–121.

6. Tronto, *Moral Boundaries;* Cancian and Oliker, *Caring and Gender,* 121.

7. Cancian and Oliker, *Caring and Gender,* 116, 120.

8. Eva Feder Kittay, "Taking Dependence Seriously: The Family and Medical Leave Act Considered in Light of the Social Organization of Dependency Work and Gender Equality," *Hypatia* 10, no. 1 (Winter 1995): 11.

9. Celia A. Conrad, "Family Allowances and Poverty among Lone Mother Families in the United States," in C. Michael Henry, ed., *Race, Poverty and Domestic Policy* (New Haven, CT: Yale University Press, 2004), 572–573; Mary Daly, *The Gender Division of Welfare: The Impact of the British and German Welfare States* (Cambridge: Cambridge University Press, 2000), 81–82; Susan Pedersen, *Family, Dependence, and the Origins of the Welfare State: Britain and France, 1914–1945* (Cambridge: Cambridge University Press, 1993), 371, 410, 411; Lou Mandin and Bruno Palier, "Country Report on France," National Reports on Welfare Reform, 1980-01, Working Papers, Welfare Reform and Management of Societal Change, University of Kent, 21, 23, available at http://www.kent.ac.uk/wramsoc/workingpapers/firstyear reports/nationalreports/francecountryreport.pdf (accessed August 20, 2009); Diane Sainsbury, *Gender, Equality and Welfare States* (Cambridge: Cambridge University Press, 1996), 86–87; Viola Desideria Burau, Hildegard Theobald, and Robert H. Blank, *Governing Home Care: A Cross-National Comparison* (Northampton, MA: Edward Elgar Publishing, 2007), 105, 107–108.

10. For example, see Paul Dickson and Thomas B. Allen, *The Bonus Army: An American Epic* (New York: Walker and Co., 2004).

11. For accounts by activists and researchers of the disability rights movement, see Paul K. Longmore and Laurie Umansky, eds., *The New Disability History: American Perspectives* (New York: New York University Press, 2001); Doris Zames Fleischer and Frieda Zames, *The Disability Rights Movement: From Charity to Confrontation* (Philadelphia: Temple University Press, 2000).

12. Andrea Cohen and Judy Willet, "Intentional Communities for Aging in Place: Consumers Taking the Lead," available at http://www.house-works .com/docs/Aging%20Today%20Article.pdf (accessed December 1, 2008); Tim Neville, "Birds of a Feather," *New York Times,* April 6, 2007, available at travel.nytimes.com/2007/04/06/travel/escapes/06retire.html (accessed December 1, 2008).

13. Carol Stack and Linda Burton, "Kinscripts: Reflections on Family, Generation, and Culture," in Evelyn Nakano Glenn, Grace Chang, and Linda Forcey, eds., *Mothering: Ideology, Experience and Agency* (New York: Routledge, 1994), 33–44.

14. Janet Finch, "Family Rights and Responsibilities," in Martin Bulmer and Anthony M. Rees, eds., *Citizenship Today: The Contemporary Relevance of T. H. Marshall* (London: UCL Press, 1996), 204; Jenny Morris, "Creating a Space for Absent Voices: Disabled Women's Experience of Receiving Assistance with Daily Living Activities," *Feminist Review* 51 (1995): 96–87; Cancian and Oliver, *Caring and Gender,* 99.

15. Finch, "Family Rights," 207.

16. Nancy Folbre, "For Love or Money—Or Both?" *Journal of Economic Perspectives* 14, no. 4 (2002): 128.

17. Margaret Radin, *Contested Commodities* (Cambridge, MA: Harvard University Press, 1996), 105.

18. Deborah Stone, "Care as We Give It, Work as We Know It," in Madonna Harrington-Meyer, ed., *Care Work: Gender, Labor and the Welfare State* (New York: Routledge, 2000), 105.

19. Quoted in Cancian and Oliker, *Caring and Gender,* 99.

20. Ibid., 155.

21. In the long term, a more universal approach will be influenced by provisions of twenty-first-century federal health care legislation, and by the likely expansion of both public and private long-term care insurance.

22. Dorothy Sue Cobble, "The Prospects for Unionization in a Service Economy," in Cameron Macdonald and Carmen Siriani, eds., *Working in a Service Economy* (Philadelphia: Temple University Press, 1996), 333–358; Service Employees International Union, "Drive to Improve L.A. Homecare Takes Big Step Forward," press release, 1999.

23. Cancian and Oliker, *Gender and Caring,* 75, 155.

24. Kittay, "Taking Dependence Seriously," 22, 23.

25. Peter S. Arno, Carol Levine, and Margaret M. Memmott, "The Economic Value of Informal Caregiving," *Health Affairs* 18, no. 2 (1999): 183, 184.

26. Calculated from U.S. Department of Labor, *Chartbook of International Labor Comparisons,* chart 2.9, available at http://www.bls.gov/fls/chartbook.htm (accessed December 16, 2009).

27. Interestingly, the U.S. Army has become a model in this regard, providing training and rewards for engaging in child care and also enforcing antidiscrimination policies and instituting a thorough comparable-worth program (in which jobs are analyzed as to the skills and responsibilities they entail so that jobs requiring comparable skills and responsibilities can be granted similar pay) to equalize pay for male and female positions. See Cancian and Oliker, *Gender and Caring,* 129–130.

Acknowledgments

The ideas and analyses in this book were enriched by interactions and exchanges with numerous colleagues and friends over many years. I can name only a relative few among those whose lives and work have inspired and sustained my work.

As always I am grateful to the Women and Work Group—Chris Bose, Myra Marx Ferree, Fran Rothstein, and Carole Turbin—and to my fellow travelers in Gender and Women's Studies and Asian American Studies at the University of California, Berkeley: Paola Bacchetta, Mel Chen, Minoo Moallem, Juana Maria Rodriguez, Charis Thompson, Barrie Thorne, Trinh Minh-ha, Catherine Ceniza Choy, Elaine Kim, Michael Omi, Khatharya Um, and Sau-ling Wong. I learned much from the philosophers, legal scholars, historians, sociologists, anthropologists, and political and policy specialists brought together at the Center for Working Families at Berkeley by co-directors Arlie Hochschild and Barrie Thorne, who created a nurturing culture of care at the Center. The initial framing of the book was unveiled at a weekend research retreat sponsored by the Center for Race and Gender at Berkeley; Paola Bachetta, Elaine Kim, Lisa Lowe, Paula Moya, Renya Ramirez, Hertha Sweet-Wong, and Ula Taylor offered warm encouragement.

Further into the project, I was fortunate to be part of a research group on work in the lives of women of color led by Sharon Harley at the University of Maryland. The culminating experience was a week-long conference at the Rockefeller Foundation Study and Conference Center at Bellagio, Italy. My sister participants—Akosua Adomako Ampofo, Carole Boyce-Davies, Elsa Barkley Brown, Akosua K. Darkwah, Nandini Gunewardena, Nancy A. Hewitt, Evelyn Hu-Dehart, Seung-kyung Kim, Maria L. Ontiveros, Mary Johnson Osirim, and Francille Wilson—reminded me of the need to attend to women's experiences and voices. I gained further transnational perspectives from participating in

251

the Colloque Internationale du Politiques du Care in Paris. I thank organizers Pascale Molinier, Patricia Paperman, and Sandra Laugier and commentators Elsa Dorlin, Daniele Kergoat, and Genevieve Cresson, and co-speakers Nina Eliasoph and Joan Tronto.

For research assistance, I thank Annie Fukushima for locating and summarizing congressional hearings on the Fair Labor Standards Act Amendments, and Marlene Harmon, reference librarian at the Boalt Hall School of Law Library, for help in tracking down hard-to-find law cases. Among those who generously shared their published and unpublished research were Eileen Boris, Grace Chang, Mignon Duffy, Jody Heyman, María de la Luz Ibarra, John Kaiser, Cameron Macdonald, Rhacel Parrenas, Katie Quan, Lynn Rivas, Dorothy Roberts, and Peggie Smith, who also wrote a brilliant amicus curiae brief for the U.S. Supreme Court hearing in the Evelyn Coke case, on which I was honored to be co-signer.

Finally, and as always, enormous gratitude to Gary Glenn for his intellectual brilliance, support, and caring. He is an astute critic of contemporary race and gender inequality and benighted social welfare policy, and he helped to hone the arguments and writing in the book. His love and that of my family—Sara Jotoku, Antonia Glenn, Patrick Glenn, Paul Nolan, Scott Horstein, and Haru Nakano—have sustained me.

Index